Diseases of bone and joints

Diseases of bone and joints

Louis Lichtenstein, M.D.

Clinical Professor of Pathology, University of California,
San Francisco; Professor Extraordinario, National University of
Mexico; Honorary Member, Spanish Orthopedic Society
(SECOT); Honorary Member, Western Orthopedic
Association; Fellow, New York Academy of Medicine; Consultant
in Pathology, Children's Hospital, San Francisco; Consultant in
Pathology, U. S. Naval Hospital, Oakland; Consultant in
Orthopaedic Pathology, St. Joseph's Hospital and
Mt. Zion Hospital and Medical Center,
San Francisco, California

With 287 illustrations

Saint Louis

The C. V. Mosby Company

1970

To all my students over the years
who have provided me with as much
stimulation as I hope
I have given them.

———————————————

Preface

For some years now I have been urged repeatedly by my colleagues to write a book that would cover skeletal disease in general, apart from neoplasms, and that might serve as a companion volume to *Bone Tumors*. If I have not done so sooner, it is because the task appeared to be so formidable, crossing as it does ever so many specialty boundary lines. Skeletal tissues are very labile, despite their mineralized structure. There is constant new bone formation and resorption in progress, even in adults, and these processes may be accelerated and otherwise thrown out of balance under certain abnormal regulatory conditions. Furthermore, as the table of contents indicates, the structure, function, and pathologic alterations of bone and joints may reflect in many obvious and subtle ways what is going on elsewhere in the body—genetic abnormalities, altered renal function, metabolic disorders, vitamin imbalances, endocrine malfunction, neurotrophic disorders, blood diseases, and many other disease states.

This monograph is intended to provide a concise yet informative comprehensive survey for basic orientation, with emphasis on pathology, and, as such, to help meet the needs of orthopedists, general surgeons, radiologists, pathologists, pediatricians, in-ternists, and other men in medicine and its allied sciences who have an interest in diseases of bone and joints, for whatever reason. It makes no pretense of being an encyclopedic treatise covering in detail every aspect of every conceivable subject in the field. That might require half a professional lifetime and, after all, teaching and consultation work are time consuming. There are relatively few existing books of comparable scope, in the English language at least, and their approach is somewhat different. In addition, I am not always in agreement with the views they express.

In the preparation of certain chapters I have perforce drawn upon the collective wisdom and published experience of my friends in internal medicine and endocrinology, some of them brilliant investigators who know far more than I do in these areas. Illustrative roentgenograms have been freely utilized as invaluable tools in graphically depicting many conditions. With few exceptions these have been selected from my own teaching files. Many of the observations on pathologic conditions are based upon articles that my associates and I have published (on such subjects as aneurysmal bone cyst, fibrous dysplasia, eosinophilic granuloma of bone, histiocytosis X, gout, hereditary ochronosis, and pigmented villonodular synovitis, among others), as well as upon unpublished data that have accrued over the past 20 years or more. Relevant physiologic, genetic, immunologic, and biochemical data have been integrated at every opportunity with clinical and pathologic findings.

Louis Lichtenstein

3903 Middlefield Rd.
Palo Alto, Calif. 94303

Contents

1 Fractures and their sequelae, 1

2 Systematized anomalies of skeletal development, 10

3 Infections of bone, 38

4 Skeletal changes in vitamin deficiencies and excesses, 60

5 Skeletal changes in endocrine disorders, 73

6 Skeletal changes in metabolic disorders, 86

7 Skeletal changes in renal disease, 100

8 Osteoporosis (osteopenia), 104

9 Skeletal changes in neurotrophic disorders, 108

10 Skeletal changes in certain blood diseases, 115

11 Paget's disease of bone (osteitis deformans), 122

12 Histiocytosis X (eosinophilic granuloma, Letterer-Siwe disease, and Schüller-Christian disease), 135

13 Chemical and radiation effects on bone, 146

14 Pathology of some common and unusual orthopedic conditions, 151

15 Disorders of synovial joints, 184

Diseases of bone and joints

Chapter 1

Fractures and their sequelae

The subject of fractures is important because of the disability that fractures may produce and because fractures constitute by far the most commonly encountered skeletal lesion.

A fracture may be defined broadly as any break in the continuity of a bone, from whatever cause. An important practical distinction is generally made between fractures that are closed (simple) and those that are open (compound) and hence prone to infection. Numerous additional qualifying designations are also employed clinically to indicate further the particular location, type, and extent of various fractures, and especially their degree of fragmentation, the direction of the break, and the displacement of the affected bone. Terms such as incomplete (Fig. 1-1), comminuted, greenstick, fissure, stress (Fig. 1-2), subperiosteal, and epiphyseal, among many others, are used, not to mention literally dozens of eponyms referring to specific situations.

A fracture through a bone area that has been weakened by some antecedent lesion is commonly referred to as a pathologic fracture; some of the major predisposing causes of this fracture will be indicated in the following discussion.

In this brief discussion emphasis will be placed upon the basic pathologic aspects of the healing of fractures in general and upon failure to achieve satisfactory bony union. For comprehensive consideration of surgical management and of the practical

Fig. 1-1. Fibrous repair of an incomplete fracture extending through articular cartilage and into subchondral bone for a short distance.

1

Fig. 1-2. Roentgenogram showing callus formation at the site of a stress fracture in a lower femur. Biopsy was done because of concern over the possibility of osteogenic sarcoma.

problems entailed in dealing effectively with special situations, the reader may have recourse to the available clinical monographs on fractures, among which the standard reference treatises of Watson-Jones and Campbell are particularly informative.

Although the healing of a fracture is a continuous process,[1] it appears to be conventional, by way of didactic exposition,[2] to postulate three distinct stages: (1) organization of hematoma at the fracture site (by granulation tissue and fibrous connective tissue), leading to so-called procallus; (2) conversion of procallus to fibrocartilaginous callus, which fills the gap be-

tween the fracture ends; and (3) replacement in turn by osseous callus, resulting in most instances in bony union. While this neat sequence is calculated to appeal to the orderly mind of the anatomist, one does not usually observe such clear-cut stages in pathologic specimens showing recent fracture. Instead, one finds the various phases of the healing of fractures—specifically, the organization of blood clots, disposal of necrotic bone debris, fibrous replacement of resorbed bone, and exuberant formation of both cartilage and bone, representing callus—going on more or less simultaneously. It would seem more realistic, therefore, to relate what happens at a fracture site in terms of actual observation rather than as a schematized hypothesis.

To interpret the sequence of events following a fracture, it is essential to be familiar with the timetable, as it were, of the changes outlined above. According to Watson-Jones and others, continuity by "granulation tissue" is achieved ordinarily within a few weeks, union by "primary callus" in 2 to 3 months, and consolidation and maturation of callus in 4 to 5 months, whereas complete restoration of structure and tubulation requires almost a year. To be sure, these estimates represent convenient averages and may need revision in any individual case, one way or the other, depending upon the location and the extent of the fracture and the age and condition of the patient, among other factors. For example, children may deposit abundant callus with surprising rapidity, to judge by adult standards. Then too, the time intervals cited do not apply to instances in which there is appreciably delayed union or eventual nonunion, for whatever reason.

The pathologic picture at the site of a fresh fracture is characterized by two cardinal features: (1) necrosis of bone of variable extent at the fracture site, reflecting loss of blood supply, and (2) hemorrhage resulting from rupture of blood vessels. Thus if one examines sections of a fracture fragment (from a patella or a head of a radius, for example) removed in the course of open repair several days after an injury, one may readily perceive that the bone is substantially if not completely dead, as evidenced by loss of osteocytes within the lacunae. It may also be found that there has been extensive extravasation of blood along the fracture line; this extends into the contiguous spongy bone for an appreciable distance. Concomitantly, there is extravasation and seepage of blood into the periosteum and adjacent soft parts, particularly the muscles, although reference to this hemorrhage as a hematoma in the conventional sense of a circumscribed tumor-like swelling may be somewhat inaccurate. Be that as it may, the presence of extensive blood clot undoubtedly helps to provide a favorable medium for relatively rapid and intensive ossification.

Also, in this connection biochemical investigations have indicated that there is a greatly increased concentration of calcium and phosphorus at a fracture site for the first several weeks at least. This increment may well be related to vascular resorption and demineralization of the fractured bone ends. Of comparable importance is the observation[3] that phosphatase activity at a fracture site becomes strikingly increased within several days and that this heightened activity persists for some 2 months.

The formation of cartilage and bone at a fracture site, constituting what is conventionally referred to as primary callus, likewise sets in relatively early, to judge by clinical as well as experimental material.[1] If one examines sections of a healing fracture in a rib, for example, several weeks after injury, one observes irregular fields of actively growing cartilage undergoing os-

Fig. 1-3. Photomicrograph of cartilaginous and bony callus at the site of a 3-week-old fracture of a rib. The callus at this stage is still relatively bulky and contains abundant cartilage.

Fig. 1-4. Photomicrograph showing abundant active formation of cartilage at a fracture site. Pathologists unfamiliar with pictures such as this are sometimes unduly concerned over the possibility of chondrosarcoma.

seous transformation intermingled with heavy-set trabeculae of new bone covered by proliferating osteoblasts. The early abundant formation of cartilage, presumably by the active cambium layer of the torn periosteum, may well be a result of local anoxia (Fig. 1-3). This cartilage component of the callus extends into the medullary cavity, where it merges with richly vascularized, young connective tissue containing organizing fibrin and bits of necrotic bone debris (Fig. 1-3). The new bone seems clearly to be of periosteal origin, for the most part, and is deposited as a tapered thick layer on the surface of the rib, extending like cantilevers to either side of the fracture line. At this stage, however, only the scaffold has been erected, as it were, while the defect in the interior has not yet been bridged by bone.

Within the next few months, barring delayed union or nonunion, internal as well as external bony union is accomplished. This is reflected pathologically in fairly complete osseous transformation of cartilage, resorption of residual necrotic bone, and condensation and remodeling of the peripheral callus. Finally reconstruction of the medullary cavity and restoration of the bone marrow (commonly referred to as tubulation) are gradually brought about. A more detailed account of this process of healing and reconstruction may be found in the lucid description of Ham in his textbook of histology.[1]

Although most appropriately treated fractures go on to uneventful solid bony union in essentially the manner described, with only minor residual disability or perhaps none at all, an appreciable number (notably, in the shaft of the tibia, the forearm bones, and the femoral neck) fails to heal for one reason or another. There are many causes of *nonunion*, some of them preventable, and much attention is devoted to them in clinical texts.

Inadequate immobilization or immobilization for too short a time is undoubtedly one of the major causes of nonunion. As Watson-Jones has strongly admonished, meticulous attention to adequate immobilization of the affected part is of the utmost importance in attaining a good result. Extensive loss of bone substance, leaving too large a defect to be successfully bridged, may be the factor responsible in some instances. Poor apposition or malposition of fracture fragments resulting from faulty surgical technique and failure to overcome distraction due to torsion and other powerful muscle stresses are also common predisposing factors. Interposition of muscle, fascia, and other soft tissues is still another. Inadequate blood supply resulting from rupture or thrombosis of nutrient vessels may result not only in nonunion but also in avascular necrosis of the affected bone (for example, of the femoral head after fracture of the neck). Excessive resorption of fractured bone ends may likewise be responsible for nonunion. Finally, old age, faulty nutrition, serious systemic disease, and a variety of other unfavorable constitutional factors may militate against the production of adequate bony callus on schedule.

In this connection, one may broadly stress these general requirements:

1. Adequate protein for osseous matrix
2. Enough vitamin C for adequate deposition of collagen (the connective tissue substratum of osteoid)
3. Sufficient vitamin D for calcification of osteoid and its conversion to bone
4. Essential concentrations of readily available calcium and phosphorus (the necessary mineral ingredients)
5. Adequate phosphatase activity for the effective utilization of calcium and phosphorus at the fracture site
6. Endocrine activity and interplay conducive to positive calcium balance and active ossification in general

The role of a local tissue inductor substance in promoting osteogenesis has been stressed by Urist, Mazet, and McLean,[4] although their inferences are drawn from transplantation studies in experimental animals.

Another important factor responsible for delayed union, and often for eventual nonunion of open or compound fractures particularly, is *infection*. The problem of healing may be enormously complicated by osteomyelitis with its sequelae of extensive vascular resorption of bone, sequestrum formation and draining sinuses, stiffness of neighboring joints, circulatory impairment of the affected part, and loss of good overlying skin. The practical obstacles entailed in coping with a comminuted infected fracture (such as of the tibia, following a motorcycle accident) are all too familiar to experienced orthopedic surgeons. By the time the infection has fully subsided, the loss of bone substance may be sufficiently great to raise a formidable problem in surgical reconstruction. It is not unusual in such cases to spend several years in futile attempts to salvage a useful lower limb.

Whatever the factors responsible for nonunion, if one examines relevant pathologic specimens removed in the course of corrective surgical procedures, one regularly observes that the gap between the fractured bone ends is filled by vascularized fibrous connective tissue (Fig. 1-5). Although this fibrous tissue is rich in capillaries and sometimes contains small inactive foci of cartilage, as a rule it shows little or no tendency to active bone formation. The impression one gains is that the process of internal bony bridging has come to an abortive standstill and that, in the absence of surgical intervention (such as grafting or shingling) calculated to stimulate osteogenesis anew, it is likely to remain dormant indefinitely. In time, cer-

5

Fig. 1-5. A, Photomicrograph of a specimen from a site of nonunion showing two fracture fragments separated by a tract of fibrous connective tissue. This is permeated by capillaries and contains an occasional small bit of inactive cartilage, but it shows no indication whatsoever of osteogenesis. **B,** Photomicrograph of another comparable specimen showing fibrous union.

Fig. 1-6. Selected field of a fracture fragment showing avascular necrosis (the lacunae are devoid of osteocytes) and beginning creeping substitution.

tain secondary changes may take place within the fibrous connective tissue at a site of nonunion. Specifically, focal deposition of fibrinoid material may be noted, as well as myxoid degeneration and cystic softening, often leading to the formation of a sinuous cleft-like space commonly referred to as a *pseudoarthrosis* or false joint. The lining of a pseudoarthrosis may actually come to resemble synovium.

The question of what happens eventually to a necrotic fracture fragment is pertinent here. Basically, this depends upon whether there is an avalaible source of blood supply, which is always an essential requisite for osseous reconstruction. Thus a loose intraarticular fracture fragment (joint body) that has no attachment to the capsule retains its dead bony core indefinitely, although it may slowly increase in size through the accretion of cartilage upon its surface. On the other hand,

a necrotic area of bone that is not displaced and that has retained its blood supply (for example, in the femoral head) undergoes reconstruction through gradual creeping replacement or substitution; that is to say, trabeculae of new bone are deposited upon the original dead bone through osteoblastic activity (Fig. 1-6). While this process of osseous reconstruction may be relatively rapid in a child (as in Legg-Perthes' disease), it is likely to be quite slow in an adult, often requiring many years for substantial repair of a sizable area.

As noted, a fracture occurring at the site of a preexisting lesion that has attenuated the bone or otherwise rendered it more vulnerable to injury is generally referred to as a *pathologic fracture*. It is not at all unusual for a break to occur in the thinned cortex overlying a bone tumor, which may be either benign or malignant. Thus the initial clinical manifestation of an enchon-

7

droma in a finger phalanx or of a nonosteo-genic fibroma in a lower limb bone may be pain referable to cortical infraction. Similarly, fracture may direct attention to a focus of metastatic carcinoma.

Fracture through the attenuated expanded cortex of a bone cyst in the metaphysis or upper shaft of a humerus is a fairly common occurrence (Fig. 1-7). A focus of eosinophilic granuloma of bone is very likely to break through the cortex rapidly and extend into the adjacent muscle tissue.

Granulomatous infections, too, may sometimes be responsible for pathologic fracture. In severe rickets and scurvy one may observe epiphyseal separation as a complication. In osteomalacia (the adult counterpart of vitamin D rickets), symmet-rical transverse fissure fractures may develop in the lower limb bones and at other sites, giving rise to the picture of Milkman's syndrome. Transverse fissure fractures may also be observed occasionally in lesions of Paget's disease, especially in the tibia. Extensively resorbed bones in hyperparathyroidism are likewise predisposed to fracture. As for the vertebral column in particular, compression fractures may be a result of any condition leading to advanced demineralization, be it metastatic carcinoma, multiple myeloma, osteoporosis, or sprue.

The articular bone ends in a neuropathic joint are particularly susceptible to multi-

Fig. 1-7. Roentgenogram showing pathologic fracture of the cortex of the neck of the femur (of a young woman, age 22) at the site of a latent solitary unicameral bone cyst.

Fig. 1-8. Another pathologic fracture through a lesion of fibrous dysplasia in the upper shaft of a femur.

ple fractures; this is true also in hereditary ochronosis, an inbred metabolic disorder. To cite still another instance in point, lesions of bone in certain of the systematized anomalies of skeletal development, especially osteogenesis imperfecta and sometimes fibrous dysplasia (Fig. 1-8), are likewise vulnerable to minor injury. Also, in marble bone disease, the affected bones, though abnormally dense, are brittle. There are undoubtedly many other conditions in which pathologic fracture may occur, but it is hardly feasible in this brief discussion to list every conceivable circumstance.

References

1. Ham, A. W.: Histology, ed. 6, Philadelphia, 1969, J. B. Lippincott Co.
2. Maximow, A. A., and Bloom, W.: A textbook of histology, ed. 9, Philadelphia, 1968, W. B. Saunders Co.
3. Botterell, E. H., and King, E. J.: Phosphatase in fractures, Lancet **228**:1267-1270, 1935.
4. Urist, M. R., Mazet, R., Jr., and McLean, F. C.: The pathogenesis and treatment of delayed union and non-union, J. Bone Joint Surg. **36A**:931-967, 1954.

General reference

Morris, J. M.: Fatigue fractures: a clinical study, Springfield, Illinois, 1967, Charles C Thomas, Publisher.

Chapter 2

Systematized anomalies of skeletal development

When one considers that there are more than 200 bones in the skeleton and that their embryologic development is inherently complex both genetically and biochemically, it is not surprising that the number of congenital anomalies of all kinds is great. With reference to the hand, for example, arachnodactyly, brachydactyly, syndactyly, hypodactyly, and polydactyly are only some of the developmental aberrations observed. Similarly, a wide range of congenital deformities is known to occur also in the foot, hip, knee, vertebral column, and skull, as well as in cther skeletal parts. Everything that may possibly go wrong apparently does so at one time or another. While these localized anomalies are of practical moment, especially to geneticists, pediatricians, and orthopedic surgeons, we are concerned here more particularly with widespread or systematized developmental disorders of the skeleton.

There are more than a dozen well-recognized, systematized developmental anomalies; there are undoubtedly many others that, because of their comparative rarity or the paucity of available biopsy material, have not yet been clearly delineated. The pertinent conditions that will be surveyed briefly in this chapter are fibrous dysplasia of bone, hereditary multiple exostosis, skeletal enchondromatosis, osteopetrosis, osteogenesis imperfecta, achondroplasia, Morquio's disease, osteopoikilosis, cleidocranial dysostosis, gargoylism, melorheostosis, progressive diaphyseal dysplasia, and monomelic medullary osteosclerosis.

Some of these conditions vary in extent and severity and, accordingly, may affect a single bone (forme fruste), several bones (which may or may not comprise a functional unit), one or more limb buds, or the major part of the skeleton. Others are universal in their skeletal effects. In several anomalies listed—fibrous dysplasia, skeletal enchondromatosis, osteogenesis imperfecta, and gargoylism—the inborn error of development, while predominantly skeletal in its impact, is genetically complex and may have its reflection in certain extraskeletal anomalies as well. In others, it is well known from study of family pedigrees that there is a significant hereditary factor. Thus the genetic defect is transmitted as a mendelian dominant in achondroplasia, cleidocranial dysostosis, osteogenesis imperfecta, and multiple exostosis. Familial incidence has also been noted in gargoylism and osteopetrosis.

As for the time of appearance of the anomalies, in some the skeletal alterations may already be clinically obvious in the neonate, as in achondroplasia, osteogenesis imperfecta, and osteopetrosis. In others the abnormalities may not become manifest for some years after birth, as in multiple exostosis, Morquio's disease, and the milder expressions of fibrous dysplasia of bone.

At the outset, a few general remarks concerning nomenclature seem to be indicated in the interest of clarity. For virtually all of the conditions under consideration, several, if not many, designations have been employed by various authors. While one of necessity must be preferred for the purpose of discussion, the more common alternative names will be mentioned for convenient orientation. I do not favor the use of eponyms, although in dealing with a disorder like Morquio's disease (in which the eponym enjoys general usage, whereas the suggested alternatives are not even well known) there is little choice.

Further, the use of vague, broad categories such as chondrodystrophy or dyschondroplasia will be avoided, since their use impedes general understanding of the conditions in question. Dyschondroplasia is another name for cartilage dysplasia, but it must be recognized that there are at least six common skeletal developmental anomalies that may be regarded as cartilage dysplasias of various types: multiple exostosis, skeletal enchondromatosis, osteopetrosis, achondroplasia, Morquio's disease, and (sometimes) fibrous dysplasia. For one to speak, therefore, of dyschondroplasia (or chondrodystrophy) without specifying the particular disorder is likely to be more confusing than helpful.

It is hardly possible within the limited scope of this monograph to describe the full picture of each of the disorders considered. (For convenient clinical orientation, the reader may have recourse to the splendidly illustrated atlas of Sir Thomas Fairbank.) In this concise survey, the emphasis will be upon the essential pathologic features, insofar as they are recognized, as a basis for better understanding of the condition. Where roentgenograms are helpful in graphic illustration, they will be freely utilized.

Fibrous dysplasia of bone

With the possible exception of hereditary multiple exostosis, fibrous dysplasia is probably the most frequently encountered anomaly of skeletal development. Considerable interest has been shown in the condition, and the pertinent literature of the past 25 years has grown too voluminous to be catalogued here.

In 1938, I directed attention to the distinctive pathologic character of the skeletal lesions and introduced the name "polyostotic fibrous dysplasia" to designate this appropriately.[1] The qualifying adjective "polyostotic" was later dropped when it became evident that often only a single bone or a portion of one bone is involved (monostotic form or forme fruste).

Such solitary foci are much more common than is generally appreciated.[2] They are encountered mainly in the ribs, the large limb bones, and the jaw and skull bones. Solitary foci are often clinically silent; they may be discovered following an injury or in the course of roentgenographic examination of the part for some other reason (Fig. 2-1). The gross and microscopic appearance of such solitary lesions is not essentially different from that of comparable lesions in cases showing more extensive involvement, and there is every reason to believe that monostotic and polyostotic lesions of fibrous dysplasia are quantitatively different expressions of the same disorder.

When more than one focus of fibrous dysplasia is present, the involved bones are likely to be solely or predominantly on one side of the body and are often confined to a single lower or upper limb bud. Occasional patients may exhibit the severe expression of the disorder in which a major part of the skeleton is affected, and the resulting deformities and disability then be-

11

Fig. 2-1. Roentgenograms illustrating the appearance of monostotic lesions of fibrous dysplasia in various common locations.

Fig. 2-2. Roentgenograms illustrating polyostotic fibrous dysplasia.

come manifest early in childhood (Fig. 2-2). The occurrence in such cases of associated extraskeletal changes, particularly blotchy cutaneous hyperpigmentation and certain endocrine abnormalities (notably pubertas praecox in females), was noted in the 1930's by Goldhamer, Borak, and Doll, McCune and Bruch,[3] and Albright and his colleagues.[4,5] The last group particularly publicized these more dramatic cases in children, presenting various extraskeletal abnormalities in addition to widespread severe skeletal alterations. In fact, this clinical picture came to be designated by many, both in the United States and abroad, as *Albright's syndrome,* although Albright himself subsequently recommended that the name "fibrous dysplasia" be generally adopted to apply to all instances of the disorder, irrespective of the severity.

In regard to those extraskeletal abnormalities, I had occasion in 1942, in a discussion of the steadily expanding literature on the subject,[6] to point out that in a number of instances hyperthyroidism, ephemeral premature skeletal growth and maturation, and cardiorenal congenital defects had also been observed. Incidentally, this survey is still useful for general orientation, as are also the excellent reviews by Falconer, Cope, and Robb-Smith,[7] Jaffe,[8,9] and others.

When one considers the condition as a whole, there is much to support the view that fibrous dysplasia has its basis in a genetically complex defect of development in which the clinical picture reflecting the skeletal lesions may be amplified at times by various extraskeletal abnormalities. The skeletal lesions result apparently from perverted activity of the bone-forming mesenchyme. This is manifested in replacement of the spongiosa and in filling of the medullary cavity of affected bone sites by a peculiar fibrous tissue in which trabeculae (or spherules or curlicues) of poorly calcified fiber bone are formed by osseous metapla-

sia (Fig. 2-3). Changus[10] has demonstrated that the dysplastic connective tissue contains abundant alkaline phosphatase, which is rather what one might expect. This osteogenic potential is not always realized, however, and some fields may be predominantly collagenous and may manifest comparatively little deposition of new bone.

In occasional instances of fibrous dysplasia, more or less prominent islands of hyaline cartilage (remote from cartilage plate regions) may also be observed (Fig. 2-3, *B*). This finding suggests a possible genetic relationship between fibrous dysplasia of bone and skeletal enchondromatosis.

In cases showing polyostotic involvement, the long bones of the lower extremity are most frequently affected, but those of the upper extremity and the skull, ribs, pelvis, phalanges, and other bones may also be involved. Extensively involved, weight-bearing bones like the femurs tend to become expanded, bowed, appreciably shortened, and otherwise deformed; they are then vulnerable to pathologic fracture (Fig. 2-2, *A*). Extensive calvarial involvement may lead eventually in some instances to Paget-like thickening (Fig. 2-2, *B*), and comparable involvement of the facial bones may occasionally give rise to a clinical picture resembling leontiasis ossea. Epiphysioid bones (carpals and tarsals) and bones preformed in membrane may likewise be affected. The aforementioned changes result, as noted, in more or less prominent widening of affected bones, thinning of their cortices, and replacement of the cancellous bone and bone marrow by a peculiar, rubbery, whitish, somewhat gritty connective tissue, which may show partial cystic softening as a secondary degenerative change, especially in lesions of long standing. At times, small nests of foam cells or foci of giant cell reaction to blood extravasation may be encountered.

By way of differential diagnosis, it should be noted that the literature records instances of adult patients with fairly extensive fibrous dysplasia of bone who were thought to have hyperparathyroidism and who were subjected to exploration for parathyroid tumor. Solitary foci, on the other hand, may be mistaken clinically for tumors and, as such, treated more vigorously than necessary, for example, by block excision (Fig. 2-1, *A*). I have observed material from instances of involvement of the maxilla in children and teen-agers in which

Fig. 2-3. Photomicrographs showing various patterns of fibrous dysplasia, as seen in biopsy specimens. **B** also presents an island of hyaline cartilage, calcified at its periphery.

Fig. 2-4. Photograph (natural size) of a portion of a maxilla in a 7-year-old boy, resected on the premise that a tumor was present. Review of the sections showed the lesion to be a focus of fibrous dysplasia.

the upper jaw was widely resected in the mistaken belief that a neoplasm was present (Fig. 2-4). Actually, the surgical removal of monostotic lesions is usually elective rather than mandatory. If such a lesion, however, is still expanding (in a jaw bone, for example), painful, cosmetically deforming, or prone to pathologic fracture, it may be desirable to curet it thoroughly and to pack the defect with bone chips.

The incidence of sarcomatous change in skeletal lesions of fibrous dysplasia should be noted. Many case reports[11] have now amply confirmed the old observation of Coley and Stewart[12] that this may happen, and these observations have been compiled

Fig. 2-5. Roentgenograms from two representative instances of hereditary multiple exostosis.

by Schwartz and Alpert.[13] Malignant change may develop without prior irradiation, it may be observed in monostotic as well as polyostotic lesions, and it apparently occurs most often in bones of the craniofacial region and in large limb bones. It should be emphasized, however, that this complication is less common than it is in Paget's disease and that its overall incidence appears to be of the order of a fraction of 1%.

Hereditary multiple exostosis
(multiple cartilaginous exostoses; diaphyseal aclasis)

Hereditary multiple exostosis is one of the best known and most common systematized anomalies of skeletal development.[14,15] Detailed information in regard to its pathologic features dates back to Virchow and von Recklinghausen. Recognition of a factor of inheritance through the study of family pedigrees goes back even further, although it was not until 1925 that the genetic pattern of hereditary transmission was fully elucidated on a large scale by Stocks and Barrington.[16] Some of the other names under which relevant case material has been reported are multiple cartilaginous exostoses, multiple exostoses, hereditary deforming chondrodysplasia, and diaphyseal aclasis. The last designation is preferred by British investigators following the lead of Keith.[17] The term "hereditary multiple exostosis" is that recommended by Jaffe,[18] whose detailed discussion of the distinctive pathologic changes of the disorder and of its clinical problems is still valuable for basic orientation.

The characteristic feature of hereditary multiple exostosis is the presence of numerous, often widespread, knobby cartilage-capped bony protrusions. These are most prominent in the metaphyseal regions of the long bones (Fig. 2-5) but may appear also on the ribs, scapulae, vertebrae, and even hand and foot bones. These osteocartilaginous exostoses apparently have their

Fig. 2-6. Roentgenogram of an involved upper limb in multiple exostosis.

basis in abnormal foci of cartilage formation by the cambium layer of the periosteum.[19] At the same time, as Keith[17] has emphasized, the ends of the affected limb bones tend to become broadened and blunted, apparently from defective remodeling by the periosteum. Severely affected patients show appreciable shortening of their limb bones, and often a characteristic bowing deformity of the forearms is noted (Fig. 2-6).

Detailed information in regard to the gross and microscopic appearance of osteocartilaginous exostoses (osteochondromas) and their manner of growth may be found in discussions by Jaffe[18] and Bethge,[20] and in Chapter 4 of my monograph, *Bone Tumors.*[21] The last deals mainly with solitary osteochondroma, which may be regarded as the common, limited expression (or forme fruste) of hereditary multiple exostosis.

An osteocartilaginous exostosis is covered by thickened fibrous periosteum, beneath which there is a cap of hyaline cartilage several millimeters in thickness (Fig. 2-7).

Fig. 2-7. Photomicrograph of an osteocartilaginous exostosis (osteochondroma) showing a portion of its cartilage cap. ($\times$ 40.)

Fig. 2-8. Roentgenogram illustrating malignant (chondrosarcomatous) change in an exostosis on the upper humerus.

The lesion grows by endochondral ossification and ceases to enlarge when its growth zone is closed off by a thin plate of bone. Subsequently, the cartilage cap tends to involute, but remnants of it may persist. These retain a latent capacity for reactivated growth, affording an explanation for the occasional development of peripheral chondrosarcoma.

The incidence of malignant (chondro-

Fig. 2-9. Roentgenograms of a case of skeletal enchodromatosis (Ollier's disease) involving a lower limb. The patient was a young adult who had been aware of the condition since early childhood. Biopsy of the expanded lower femur failed to show evidence of malignant change.

sarcomatous) change in multiple exostosis through activated growth of the cartilage caps of one or more protuberances is sufficiently high to be of some concern (Fig. 2-8). A precise long-term statistical estimate of this hazard is not available, but it apparently exceeds 10%. In dealing with solitary exostoses, on the other hand, this complication is seldom encountered, and its incidence is probably less than 1%.

Skeletal enchondromatosis (*Ollier's disease*)

In skeletal enchondromatosis, central hyaline cartilage tumors are found in multiple sites. Clinical manifestations of this disease often appear early in childhood, although no hereditary factor has been demonstrated. The skeletal lesions are occasionally associated with hemangiomas of the skin (so-called Maffucci's syndrome). An informative account of the condition may be found in a survey of some eighteen instances by Carleton, Elkington, Greenfield, and Robb-Smith.[22] These authors called attention also to the incidence of anomalies other than vascular hamartomas—vitiligo (in two instances) and facial asymmetry (in six). Another well-documented report is that of Hunter and Wiles,[23] which is useful for its extensive bibliography of the older literature.

Depending upon the severity of the condition, the enchondromas may be confined to the bones of a single digit, to several or all of the digits of one or both hands, or to the bones of a single limb (usually a lower limb); or, if more extensive, they may involve many bones in both upper and lower limbs (Figs. 2-10 and 2-11). With widespread skeletal involvement, one often observes unilateral or predominantly unilateral distribution; these instances are often referred to as *Ollier's disease*. There is also a strong tendency to appreciable, if not marked, shortening of affected limbs, much more so than is usually observed in fibrous dysplasia. The areas of cartilage

Fig. 2-10. Skeletal enchondromatosis involving the large limb bones of both lower extremities in a child.

Fig. 2-11. A, Extensive involvement of an ulna in enchondromatosis. Some of the hand bones (not shown) were also affected. B, Skeletal enchondromatosis (Ollier's disease) affecting the bones of a hand.

A

B

growth may be limited to the ends of the long bones or may involve the entire shaft. These areas present roentgenographically as peculiar, broadened, rarefied defects (Fig. 2-9). As a rule there is little tendency to calcific stippling or ossification before adolescence. For further details of the roentgenographic picture, the reader is referred to the exquisite illustrations in Fairbank's atlas.[14]

If one examines a biopsy of an individual lesion in skeletal enchondromatosis, it appears more cellular, as a rule, than a solitary enchondroma. This reflects a greater growth potential, and so it is not unusual to observe malignant change during adolescence or early adult life. Thus, of the eighteen cases surveyed by Carleton and his associates,[22] sarcomatous change had occurred in four, and in three others this was "possibly true." While statistically valid estimates are difficult to arrive at, it is obvious that the hazard of chondrosarcoma in patients with skeletal enchondromatosis, even of moderate extent, is sufficiently great so that one has to be constantly on the alert for it.[21] The grotesque pictures in the older literature of patients with enchondromatosis exhibiting large protruding cartilage tumor masses on the hands, feet, or other sites furnish a striking demonstration of the spontaneous tendency to malignant change.

Osteopetrosis *(marble bone disease; Albers-Schönberg disease; osteosclerosis fragilis)*

As its name implies, osteopetrosis is characterized by abnormal density of most or all of the bones of the skeleton, as first described by the German radiologist, Albers-Schönberg[24] in 1904. It was Karshner,[25] a radiologist at the Children's Hospital in Los Angeles, who in 1926 proposed the commonly employed designation "osteopetrosis." As in many of the other skeletal anomalies, a familial and hereditary tendency has been noted.

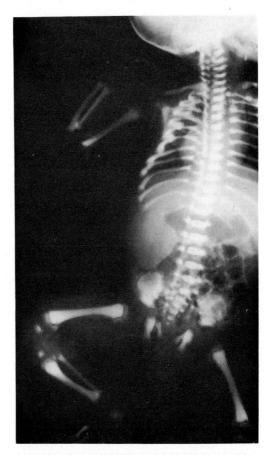

Fig. 2-12. Roentgenogram of an entire skeleton affected by osteopetrosis (marble bone disease) at 7 months of age.

The severity of osteopetrosis may vary within rather wide limits. Milder forms are not incompatible with longevity. In the severest expression, on the other hand, death may ensue in fetal life before term (Fig. 2-12). Children with outspoken involvement who survive may ultimately develop myelophthisic anemia (from encroachment of the compacted densified spongiosa upon the myeloid marrow) and hepatosplenomegaly (reflecting pronounced compensatory extramedullary hematopoiesis). Abnormal thickening and density of the base of the skull and sometimes of the facial and maxillary bones may be responsible for optic atrophy, facial palsy, and, occasionally, other neurologic manifestations. Since affected dense bones may also be brittle, a tendency to fractures may be a prominent feature in some cases. Occasionally, osteomyelitis or coxitis may develop, as well as other manifestations of infection.

The roentgenographic recognition of the condition is not usually difficult. In addition to widespread striking radiopacity of affected bones, there is a tendency to clubbing of the metaphyses of limb bones and to the development of transverse bands of varying density producing a zebra-like effect (Fig. 2-12). The only other conditions that might conceivably be considered by way of differential diagnosis are heavy metal poisoning, endemic fluorosis, and (in adults) sclerosing carcinoma extensively metastatic to the skeleton.

Pathologically, affected bones appear whitish and obviously dense. They may be substantially solid as a result of partial obliteration of the medullary cavity and fibrosis of the residual marrow. Microscopic examination of such bones from dead neonates show the presence of persistent cores of cartilage within spongy trabeculae even at a great distance from the plate regions, pointing to a defect in the normal mechanism of resorption and remodeling (Fig. 2-13). Deposition of new bone upon these unreconstructed dense trabeculae would seem to afford an adequate explanation for the abnormal bone density characterizing the disorder.

Osteogenesis imperfecta
(fragilitas ossium; brittle bones; osteopsathyrosis; Lobstein's syndrome; van der Hoeve's syndrome)

Osteogenesis imperfecta is one of the more complex developmental anomalies and is characterized in fully developed cases by morphologic alterations in the

Fig. 2-13. Photomicrograph from a case of osteopetrosis showing unresorbed cartilage cores within spongy trabeculae (at a considerable distance from the plate region).

Fig. 2-14. Photographs showing the striking deformities and stunting of stature that may ensue in severe osteogenesis imperfecta.

skeletal tissues, the eye (sclera), and the skin. The complete clinical syndrome is featured essentially by multiple fractures, blue sclerae, deafness, and loose-jointedness, as well as by other related manifestations such as scoliosis, dwarfism, hernia, "thin skin," and stunting and discoloration of the teeth, especially the lower incisors.[14,26] Abnormal aminoaciduria (familial) and low serum creatinine and uric acid levels have also been noted.[27] The disorder may be inherited from either parent and may be traced back through several generations.

The condition apparently results from a specific defect in connective tissue development or maturation. The studies of Follis[28,29] have demonstrated failure of

Fig. 2-15. Roentgenogram showing healing and recent fractures in lower limb bones of a child with osteogenesis imperfecta.

23

argyrophilic reticulin fibrils in the corium to become transformed to adult collagen fibers. Presumably a comparable defect is present in the connective tissue of the sclerae, joints, and other affected structures. The essential change in the skeleton predisposing to delicate, bent, and otherwise deformed bones prone to fracture (Figs. 2-15 and 2-16) is deficient formation of bone by osteoblasts, both in the periosteum and at sites of endochondral ossification (Fig. 2-17).

Severely affected fetuses (*osteogenesis imperfecta fetalis*) may die at birth,[30] or the infant may survive only a few days or

Fig. 2-16. Roentgenogram showing strikingly thinned and otherwise deformed bones in the leg of a patient with osteogenesis imperfecta.

Fig. 2-17. Photomicrographs of a tibia and rib respectively from an instance of osteogenesis imperfecta congenita illustrating deficient formation of bone, both in the cortex and at the epiphyseal cartilage plates.

weeks, although multiple fractures at birth are not incompatible with survival. In such subjects, so-called caput membranaceum with multiple wormian bones may be observed in the calvarium.[26] According to Stern,[31] recessive lethal or sublethal alleles are responsible for these severe cases with multiple fractures before birth.

Osteogenesis imperfecta tarda is a term sometimes used to designate the condition in which there is a delay in the appearance of fractures, for example, in a child with

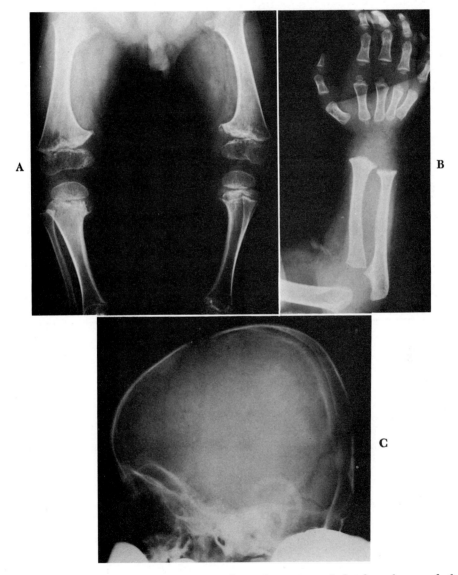

Fig. 2-18. **A,** Roentgenogram showing striking shortening of the long bones of the lower limbs in a child with achondroplasia. **B,** Roentgenogram illustrating so-called trident hand in an achondroplastic child. **C,** The skull in the same patient showing a large calvarium, wth distinct foreshortening of the base (which is largely preformed in cartilage).

blue sclerotics who does not sustain the first of many fractures until the age of 7. For that matter, blue sclerotics may be present in members of affected families without concomitant bone changes; this is ascribed by Stern[31] to a dominant gene with incomplete penetrance. The number of fractures sustained varies greatly from case to case, but in severe instances there may be as many as 100 or more. After the onset of puberty one may anticipate fewer fractures. These fractures tend to heal readily, and occasionally the callus may be so abundant as to give rise to tumor-like excrescences radiographically simulating osteogenic sarcoma. Among other skeletal changes present in many but by no means all affected patients are otosclerosis leading to progressive deafness in those who survive past 20 years of age, scoliosis (which is often severe), broadening of the skull with bulging in the temporal regions,

and dwarfing of stature in the most severe cases (Fig. 2-14).

Achondroplasia (*chondrodystrophic dwarfism; chondrodystrophia fetalis; micromelia*)

Achondroplasia results from inadequacy of cartilage cell proliferation and premature closure of the growth plates of bones preformed in cartilage. It is characterized clinically by dwarfism of the short limb type associated with a large head and, in many cases, so-called trident hands (Fig. 2-18). It is the most common type of dwarfism and perhaps the most ancient—the traditional court jester is gone, but the circus dwarf lingers on. The relative frequency of the condition may be judged from the fact that Caffey[32] observed as many as forty-three cases at Babies Hospital in New York in the course of some 15 years. Meticulously compiled family pedigrees indicate that the

Fig. 2-19. Photomicrograph showing failure of cartilage proliferation and endochondral ossification, with premature closure of the plate in a young achondroplastic subject.

condition results genetically from a dominant mutation that may be transmitted to all succeeding generations.[31] Many severely affected fetuses die in utero or soon after birth (which is often premature). On the other hand, survivors may live to an advanced age and be singularly sturdy and robust.

As noted, it is particularly the bones preformed in cartilage that are foreshortened. Thus the size of the trunk and head of affected patients is not appreciably reduced, but the limbs are very short (like those of a dachshund). Also, since many of the bones at the base of the skull develop from cartilage anlage (in contradistinction to the calvarial vault, which is preformed in membrane), one observes characteristically a sunken bridge of the nose and foreshortening of the base of the skull (Fig. 2-18, *C*).

Available pathologic studies,[33-35] some of them quite old, show that failure of normal ossification of long bones is apparent in the fetus as early as 2 to 3 months and that the large limb bones especially may be strikingly foreshortened. There appears to be a relative aplasia of cartilage at the ends of the bones, and growth of the cartilage cells of the epiphysis is disorderly. More particularly, there is an absence of a normal orderly zone of provisional calcification, leading to premature closure of epiphyseal cartilage plates (Fig. 2-19).

Morquio's disease *(chondroosteodystrophy [Morquio-Brailsford type]; eccentro-osteochondrodysplasia [Morquio]; osteochondrodystrophia deformans)*

Morquio's disease is one of the more unusual anomalies of skeletal development; only a limited number of cases have been recorded since Morquio's account[36] in 1929. Its manifestations[36-40] apparently result from a congenital defect in the ossification and development of epiphyses. A tendency to familial incidence has been demonstrated in relevant pedigrees[36]; Jacobsen,[39] for example, has noted the incidence of the disorder in twenty members of a family group followed for five generations. There is a paucity of available pathologic data, although there is some evidence to suggest that affected epiphyses manifest anomalous eccentric centers of ossification, fusion of which leads eventually to deformity.

Morquio's disease is characterized clinically and radiographically by stunting of stature, flattening or shallowness of the vertebral bodies (universal vertebra plana), marked kyphosis, sometimes angular increase of the spinal curve at the dorsolumbar junction, and progressive changes in the articular bone ends, notably in the femoral head and acetabulum (Figs. 2-20 and 2-21). Although roentgenographic changes may be present in infancy,[41] the developmental error is usually not apparent until the affected child begins to walk, and sometimes not until the age of 4 or later. The whole skeleton may be affected to a varying extent, except for bones of the skull and face. Intelligence may be normal, in contrast to gargoylism, from which Morquio's disease must be distinguished. A subject with the fully developed disorder presents, as Fairbank[14] has aptly stated, as a "round-back, knock-kneed, flat-footed child who stands with hips and knees flexed (crouch), head thrust forward and sunk between high shoulders, and walking with a waddling duck-like gait." There is often stiffness of the hip joints, less often of other joints, although the ligaments at the joints may show increased laxity.

From a biochemical standpoint, an appreciable number of articles have appeared in recent years suggesting that Morquio's disease (like gargoylism and Morquio-Ullrich disease) may reflect an abnormality of mucopolysaccharide metabolism. This literature has been surveyed by Robins, Stevens, and Linker,[41] who directed attention particularly to the abnormal urinary

Fig. 2-20. Roentgenograms showing skeletal abnormalities in the spine and hip joints of a child, age 6, with Morquio's disease.

Fig. 2-21. Skeletal alterations in an upper extremity, including the hand, of another 6-year-old child with Morquio's disease.

excretion of keratosulfate and the finding of acid mucopolysaccharide cytoplasmic granules in leukocytes (Reilly bodies). It may well be, as Robins and his associates intimate, that there is a small family of related, and sometimes overlapping, hereditary disorders of mucopolysaccharide metabolism resulting from specific enzyme defects that are characterized chiefly by bone and joint abnormalities. Considerably more information is required, however, to establish this concept firmly and to clarify the possible interrelationship of these disorders.

Osteopoikilosis *(spotty bones; osteopathia condensans disseminata)*

Osteopoikilosis is one of the less common anomalies of skeletal development.[42,43] It is a pathologic curiosity characterized by the presence of small, spotty dense bone islands[44] mainly within the limb bones, including those of the hands and feet (Fig.

Fig. 2-22. Roentgenogram showing spotty enostoses in the foot bones in osteopoikilosis.

Fig. 2-23. Roentenogram showing the anomalous vertical striations seen in Voorhoeve's disease.

2-22). These enostoses do not give rise to any apparent clinical symptoms. Familial incidence of this disorder has been noted. I have observed an unusual instance in which osteopoikilosis was associated with vertical striations in affected bones (so-called Voorhoeve's disease[45]; Fig. 2-23).

Cleidocranial dysostosis

Cleidocranial dysostosis is a well-known but rather uncommon congenital anomaly characterized by deficient formation of one or both clavicles, especially at the outer ends, associated with delayed and imperfect ossification of the calvarium (Fig. 2-24). Clinical reports of the condition date back as far as 1898.[46] In some instances there may be other developmental abnormalities as well. For detailed consideration of these unusual manifestations, the reader is referred to informative reviews of the subject by Fitzwilliams,[47] Fitchet,[48] and Soule.[49]

The hereditary and familial incidence of cleidocranial dysostosis has been well documented, and in particular, Stocks and Barrington[16] pointed out that in more than half of the cases collected the condition was inherited from one or the other parent.

29

Fig. 2-24. Photographs and roentgenograms illustrating skeletal alterations in cleido-cranial dysostosis.

Gargoylism *(Hurler's syndrome; Hurler-Pfaundler disease; dysostosis multiplex; lipochondrodystrophy)*

Gargoylism is another hereditary (familial) disorder about which we have learned a great deal in recent years. It is rather serious in its implications,[14,50-52] and many affected subjects fail to survive beyond the period of completion of growth. According to McKusick[26] there are two genotypes of gargoylism. The more frequent form, inherited as an autosomal recessive trait, is almost always accompanied by clouding of the cornea and tends to be more rapid and severe in its evolution. In the less frequent, sex-linked recessive

30

Fig. 2-25. **A,** The skull of a young child with gargoylism. **B,** Skull changes in gargoylism of child at age 10.

form, clouding of the cornea probably never occurs and the patient may live to an older age (the twenties or even later).

The condition apparently represents a peculiar lipoglycoprotein storage disease[53-58] in which the whole body, not just the skeletal structures, becomes overloaded with mucopolysaccharides, probably in chemical combination with polypeptides. This material is deposited in the central nervous system (particularly in the meninges, nerve cells, and ganglion cells), the cardiovascular and reticuloendothelial structures, and the endocrine glands, as well as the bones. As Meyer and his associates[56] have demonstrated, large amounts of sulfated mucopolysaccharides are excreted in the urine of such patients as chondroitin sulfate B and/or heparitin sulfate. The abnormal accumulation of these substances is presumably caused by a specific gene disturbance, which in turn causes an enzymatic defect, although the precise

Fig. 2-26. Skeletal alterations in gargoylism in an 18 year old.

metabolic pathway blocked is not yet known.

Clinically, the fully developed disorder is characterized by stunting of stature (dwarfism), some shortening of the limbs (micromelia), heavy grotesque facies (large head, eyes set wide apart, bridge of the nose depressed, and, occasionally, hydrocephalus), corneal opacity, deafness, mental deficiency, marked dorsolumbar kyphosis, and distension of the abdomen from hepatosplenomegaly. Other features that may be noted are limited motion in the joints, umbilical hernia, hirsutism, and clawed hands.

The roentgenographic reflections of the skeletal alterations have been sufficiently well documented[59,60] to permit their ready recognition (Figs. 2-25 and 2-26). For detailed information in regard to the pathologic changes the reader may have recourse to the valuable paper by Lindsay and his associates[55] reporting the findings in some eight autopsied cases, supplemented by additional biopsy material.

Melorheostosis (*Léri type of osteopetrosis; osteosi eburnizzante monomelica*[61])

Melorheostosis is a comparatively rare skeletal anomaly usually confined to a single limb bud, though it is sometimes more extensive. The affected bones show irregular linear, streaky, or flowing hyperostosis on their external surfaces (reminiscent of the flow of melted candle wax).[61-66] When an upper extremity is affected, the bones of the contiguous shoulder girdle may also be involved; similarly, with involvement of a lower limb, the ipsilateral iliac bone may likewise be transformed. Gradually increasing pain, often associated with stiffness and deformity of the affected region, is the usual clinical manifestation. Léri and Joanny[64] are generally credited with the first clinical report of this remarkable condition. Subsequently many other relevant papers appeared, both in the United States and abroad. The total number of cases in the literature as of 1963 was tallied at 131.[66] In 80% of these only a single limb was affected; in the remainder there was involvement of more than one limb and/or other bones, particularly the skull, vertebrae, and ribs.

The onset of the condition in childhood, its slow evolution, and its monomelic or unilateral localization strongly suggest that it represents a congenital developmental anomaly. The limited number of biopsy specimens examined have confirmed the presence of marked abnormal condensation or sclerosis of the affected bone but no other consistent distinctive alteration. The new bone formation is predominantly periosteal in origin and only in part endosteal. There may also be paraarticular bone deposits in advanced cases that may

be responsible for pain and limitation of motion.

Progressive diaphyseal dysplasia (*Engelmann's disease; osteopathia hyperostotica [sclerotisans] multiplex infantilis; hereditary multiple diaphyseal sclerosis*)

Progressive diaphyseal dysplasia is another uncommon skeletal developmental anomaly whose manifestations have been clarified in comparatively recent years. The name currently favored to designate the disorder is that introduced by Neuhauser and his associates[67] in 1948, although earlier case reports[68,69] date back to the 1920's. The pertinent literature was surveyed in 1956 by Griffiths,[70] who accepted some twenty-two cases as instances in point. Additional observations of interest were published in 1958 by Mikity and Jacobson[71] (who followed a patient for fully 22 years) and in 1964 by Clausen and Loop.[72]

The disorder is characterized roentgenographically by symmetrical sclerosis and fusiform widening of the shafts of the long bones, and often by thickening of the skull, especially at its base. Other bones (ribs, scapulae, pelvis, clavicles, hands, and feet) are infrequently involved. The condition manifests itself in childhood and may lead to physical underdevelopment, pains in the extremities, abnormal waddling gait, occasional deformities, fatigability, and weakness. The available reports indicate a tendency to progression of varying extent in childhood, but not necessarily in adult life. Presumably, some gene defect is responsible for this peculiar anomaly, as Griffiths[70] has suggested, although its pattern of hereditary transmission has not as yet been fully elucidated.[72]

Biopsies of affected limb bones in an appreciable number of instances[70-73] have indicated that the strikingly thickened bone results from endosteal and subperiosteal new bone deposition; this encroaches upon the marrow cavity, as one might expect

33

from the roentgenograms. Apart from its abnormal density, the structure of the new bone does not appear particularly unusual. For detailed study of these pathologic changes one may refer to the paper by Cohen and States,[74] who had occasion to examine a subject at autopsy.

Monomelic medullary osteosclerosis

Monomelic medullary osteosclerosis is still another comparatively rare developmental anomaly in which the bones of a single lower limb bud come to show a peculiar internal or medullary sclerosis— something like melorheostosis turned outside-in. The condition was described by Horwitz[75] in 1941, and Sotelo-Ortiz[76] in 1954 also reported a case in an 11-year-old girl who manifested unequal leg length and valgus deformity requiring surgical correction (Fig. 2-27). It is quite possible, as Sotelo-Ortiz pointed out, that additional instances have been recorded or compiled under the head of melorheostosis because their distinctive character was not recognized.

Histologically, as Horwitz indicated,[75] there is replacement of the normal spongiosa by densely sclerotic bone of unusual architecture, made up of compact, irregular segments of immature and adult bone arranged in bizarre pattern.

Other anomalies

In addition to the well-defined systematized anomalies of skeletal development already considered, there are a number of rarely observed additional disorders of which too little is known at present to serve as a basis for comprehensive discussion. Among these are *metaphyseal dysostosis* (Merk Jansen[77]), which leads to a rare form of dwarfism; *familial metaphyseal dysplasia* (Bakwin-Krida[78]), which results in symmetrical enlargement of one or both ends of the shafts of the long bones; *dysplasia epiphysealis multiplex* (Jansen-Fairbank[14]), characterized by mottled density

Fig. 2-27. Roentgenogram of a tibia showing peculiar medullary osteosclerosis, from the case reported by Sotelo-Ortiz.

and irregularity of affected epiphyses, dwarfism, and stubby digits; and *dysplasia epiphysealis punctata* (Fairbank[14,79]), manifested in stippled or speckled epiphyses. For the limited information available in regard to these and some other rare anomalies, the reader is referred again to the valuable atlas of Sir Thomas Fairbank.

References

1. Lichtenstein, L.: Polyostotic fibrous dysplasia, Arch. Surg. **36**:874, 1938.
2. Schlumberger, H. G.: Fibrous dysplasia of single bones (monostotic fibrous dysplasia), Mil. Surg. **99**:504, 1946.
3. McCune, D. J., and Bruch, H.: Osteodystrophia fibrosa; report of case in which condition was combined with precocious puberty, pathologic pigmentation of skin and hyperthyroidism, Amer. J. Dis. Child. **52**:734, 1936; ibid. **54**:806, 1937.
4. Albright, F., Butler, A. M., Hampton, A. O., and Smith, P.: Syndrome characterized by osteitis fibrosa disseminata, areas of pigmen-

tation and endocrine dysfunction, with precocious puberty in females; report of 5 cases, New Eng. J. Med. **216:**272, 1937.

5. Albright, F., Scoville, W. B., and Sulkowitch, H. W.: Syndrome characterized by osteitis fibrosa disseminata, areas of pigmentation, and gonadal dysfunction, Endocrinology **22:**411, 1938.

6. Lichtenstein, L., and Jaffe, H. L.: Fibrous dysplasia of bone: a condition affecting one, several or many bones, the graver cases of which may present abnormal pigmentation of the skin, premature sexual development, hyperthyroidism or still other extra-skeletal abnormalities, Arch. Path. **33:**777, 1942.

7. Falconer, M. A., Cope, C. L., and Robb-Smith, A.: Fibrous dysplasia of bone with endocrine disorders and cutaneous pigmentation (Albright's disease), Quart. J. Med. **11:**121, 1942.

8. Jaffe, H. L.: Fibrous dysplasia of bone, a disease entity and specifically not an expression of neurofibromatosis, J. Mount Sinai Hosp. **12:**364, 1945.

9. Jaffe, H. L.: Fibrous dysplasia of bone, Bull. N. Y. Acad. Med. **22:**588, 1946.

10. Changus, G. W.: Osteoblastic hyperplasia of bone: a histochemical appraisal of fibrous dysplasia of bone, Cancer **10:**1157, 1957.

11. Perkinson, N. B., and Higinbotham, N. L.: Osteogenic sarcoma arising in polyostotic fibrous dysplasia: report of a case, Cancer **8:**396, 1955.

12. Coley, B. L., and Stewart, F. W.: Bone sarcoma in polyostotic fibrous dysplasia, Ann. Surg. **121:**872, 1945.

13. Schwartz, D. T., and Alpert, M.: The malignant transformation of fibrous dysplasia, Amer. J. Med. Sci. **247:**350, 1964.

14. Fairbank, H. A. T.: An atlas of general affections of the skeleton, Edinburgh, 1951, E. & S. Livingstone Ltd.

15. Ollier, L.: Lyon Méd. **88:**484, 1898.

16. Stocks, P., and Barrington, A.: Hereditary disorders of bone development, University of London, Francis Galton Laboratory for National Eugenics, Memoir 22, 1925.

17. Keith, A.: J. Anat. **54:**101, 1920.

18. Jaffe, H. L.: Hereditary multiple exostosis, Arch. Path. **36:**335, 1943.

19. Müller, E.: Beitr. Path. Anat. **57:**232, 1913.

20. Bethge, J. F. J.: Hereditäre multiple Exostosen und ihre pathogenetische Deutung, Arch. Orthop. Unfallchir. **54:**667-696, 1963.

21. Lichtenstein, L.: Bone tumors, ed. 3, St. Louis, 1965, The C. V. Mosby Co.

22. Carleton, A., Elkington, J. St. C., Greenfield,

J. G., and Robb-Smith, A. H. T.: Maffucci's syndrome (dyschondroplasia with haemangiomata), Quart. J. Med. **35:**203, 1942.

23. Hunter, D., and Wiles, P.: Dyschondroplasia (Ollier's disease), with report of a case, Brit. J. Surg. **22:**507, 1935.

24. Albers-Schönberg, H.: Münchener Med. Wschr. **51:**365, 1904.

25. Karshner, R. G.: Amer. J. Roentgen. **16:**405, 1926.

26. McKusick, V. A.: Hereditary disorders of connective tissue, Bull. N. Y. Acad. Med. **35:**143-156, 1959.

27. Chowers, I., Czaczkes, J. W., Ehrenfeld, E. N., and Landau, S.: Familial aminoaciduria in osteogenesis imperfecta, J.A.M.A. **181:**771, 1962.

28. Follis, R. H., Jr.: Osteogenesis imperfecta congenita: a connective tissue diathesis, J. Pediat. **41:**713, 1952.

29. Follis, R. H., Jr.: Maldevelopment of the corium in the osteogenesis imperfecta syndrome, Bull. Johns Hopk. Hosp. **93:**225, 1953.

30. Hreno, A., and Haust, M. D.: Osteogenesis imperfecta congenita, J. Pediat. **62:**908, 1963.

31. Stern, C.: Principles of human genetics, San Francisco, 1949, W. H. Freeman & Co., Publishers.

32. Caffey, J.: In Brennemann's practice of pediatrics, vol. 4, Hagerstown, Maryland, 1957, W. F. Prior, pp. 1-22.

33. Hecktoen, L.: Anatomical study of short-limbed dwarf, with special reference to osteogenesis imperfecta and chondrodystrophia foetalis, Amer. J. Med. Sci. **125:**751, 1903.

34. Hughes Jones, E. W. A.: Studies in achondroplasia, J. Anat. **66:**565, 1932.

35. Kaufmann, E.: Die Chondrodystrophia hyperplastica, Beitr. Path. Anat. **13:**32, 1893.

36. Morquio, L.: Sur une forme de dystrophie osseuse familiale, Arch. Méd. Enf. **32:**139, 1929.

37. Brailsford, J. F.: Chondro-osteodystrophy: roentgenographic and clinical features of child with dislocation of vertebrae, Amer. J. Surg. **7:**404, 1929.

38. Einhorn, N. H., Moore, J. R., and Rowntree, L. G.: Osteochondrodystrophia deformans (Morquio's disease): observations at autopsy in 1 case, Amer. J. Dis. Child. **72:**536, 1946.

39. Jacobsen, A. W.: Hereditary osteochondrodystrophia deformans: family with twenty members affected in five generations, J.A.M.A. **113:**121, 1939.

40. Pohl, J. F.: Chondro-osteodystrophy (Morquio's disease), J. Bone Joint Surg. **12:**187, 1939.

41. Robins, M. M., Stevens, H. F., and Linker,

A.: Morquio's disease: an abnormality of mucopolysaccharide metabolism, J. Pediat. **62**:881, 1963.

42. Albers-Schönberg, H.: Eine Seltene, bisher nicht bekannte Struktur-anomalie des Skelettes, Fortschr. Roentgenstr. **23**:174, 1915.

43. Newcomet, W. S.: Spotted bones, Amer. J. Roentgen. **22**:460, 1929.

44. Schmorl, G.: Anatomische Befunde bei Einen Falle von Osteopoikilie, Fortsch. Roentgenstr. **44**:1, 1931.

45. Voorhoeve, N.: L'image radiologique non encore décrite d'une anomalie du squelette, Acta Radiol. **3**:407, 1924.

46. Marie, P., and Sainton, P.: Observation d'hydrocéphalie heréditaire (père et fils) par via de développement du crane et du cerveau, Bull. Soc. Méd. Hôp. Paris **14**:706, 1897; ibid. **15**:436, 1898.

47. Fitzwilliams, D. C. L.: Lancet, **2**:1466, 1910.

48. Fitchet, S. M.: Cleidocranial dysostosis, hereditary and familial, J. Bone Joint Surg. **11**:838, 1929.

49. Soule, A. B., Jr.: Mutational dysostosis (cleidocranial dysostosis), J. Bone Joint Surg. **28**:81, 1946.

50. Engle, D.: Dysostosis multiplex; Pfaundler-Hurler syndrome—report of 2 cases, Arch. Dis. Child. **14**:217, 1939.

51. Harvey, R. M.: Hurler-Pfaundler syndrome (gargoylism), Amer. J. Roentgen. **48**:732, 1942.

52. Hunter, C.: A rare disease in two brothers, Proc. Roy. Soc. Med. **10**:104-116, 1917.

53. Klenk, E.: The pathological chemistry of the developing brain. In Waelsch, H., editor: Biochemistry of the developing nervous system, New York, 1955, Academic Press Inc., pp. 397-410.

54. Kobayashi, N.: Acid mucopolysaccharide granules in the glomerular epithelium in gargoylism, Amer. J. Path. **35**:591, 1959.

55. Lindsay, S., Reilly, W. A., Gotham, T. J., and Skahen, R.: Gargoylism: II, study of pathologic lesions and clinical review of 12 cases, Amer. J. Dis. Child. **76**:239, 1948.

56. Meyer, K., Grumbach, M. M., Linker, A., and Hoffman, P.: Excretion of sulfated mucopolysaccharides in gargoylism (Hurler's syndrome), Proc. Soc. Exp. Biol. Med. **97**:275-279, 1958.

57. Meyer, K., and Hoffman, P.: Hurler's syndrome, Arthritis Rheum. **4**:552, 1961.

58. Tuthill, C. R.: Juvenile amaurotic idiocy; marked adventitial growth associated with skeletal malformation and tuberculomas, Arch. Neurol. Psychiat. **32**:198, 1934.

59. Ellis, R. W. B., Sheldon, W., and Capon, N.

B.: Gargoylism (chondro-osteo-dystrophy, corneal opacities, hepatosphenomegaly, and mental deficiency), Quart. J. Med. **5**:119-139, 1936.

60. Hurler, G.: Über einen Typ Multiplex Abartungen, vorwiegend am Skelettsystem, Z. Kinderheilh. **24**:220, 1920.

61. Putti, V.: L'osteosi eburnizzante monomelica, Chir. Orgagni Mov. **11**:335, 1927.

62. Franklin, E. L., and Matheson, I.: Melorheostosis: report of case with review of literature, Brit. J. Radiol. **15**:185, 1942.

63. Kraft, E.: Melorheostosis Léri; flowing hyperostosis of single extremity, report of 2 cases, J.A.M.A. **98**:705, 1932.

64. Léri, A., and Joanny, S.: Une affection non décrite des os: hyperostose "en coulée" sur toute le longeur d'un membre ou "melorhéostose," Bull. Soc. Méd. Hôp. Paris **46**:1141-1145, 1922.

65. Lewin, P., and MacLeod, S. B.: Osteosclerosis with distribution suggesting that of ulnar nerve, unclassified bone condition, J. Bone Joint Surg. **7**:968, 1925.

66. Morris, J. M., Samilson, R. L., and Corley, C. L.: Melorheostosis: review of the literature and report of an interesting case with a nineteen-year follow-up, J. Bone Joint Surg. **45-A**:1191, 1963. (Contains extensive bibliography.)

67. Neuhauser, E. B. D., Schwachman, H., Wittenborg, M., and Cohen, J.: Progressive diaphyseal dysplasia, Radiology **51**:11-22, 1948.

68. Camurati, M.: Di un raro caso di osteite simmetrica ereditaria degli arti inferori, Chir. Orgagni Mov. **6**:662-665, 1922.

69. Engelmann, G.: Ein Fall von Osteopathia hyperostotica (sclerotisans) multiplex infantilis, Fortschr. Roentgenstr. **39**:1101-1106, 1929.

70. Griffiths, D. W.: Engelmann's disease, J. Bone Joint Surg. **38-B**:312-326, 1956.

71. Mikity, V. G., and Jacobson, G.: Progressive diaphyseal dysplasia (Engelmann's disease): report of a case with twenty-two years follow-up, J. Bone Joint Surg. **40-A**:206-210, 1958.

72. Clausen, D. K., and Loop, J. W.: Progressive diaphyseal dysplasia (Engelmann's disease), J. Bone Joint Surg. **46-A**:143, 1964.

73. Mottram, M. E., and Hill, H. H.: Diaphyseal dysplasia: report of a case, Amer. J. Roentgen. **95**:162, 1965.

74. Cohen, J., and States, J. D.: Progressive diaphyseal dysplasia: report of a case with autopsy findings, Lab. Invest. **5**:492-508, 1956.

75. Horwitz, T.: Monomelic medullary osteo-

sclerosis of unknown etiology, Radiology **36:** 343, 1941.

76. Sotelo-Ortiz, F.: Monomelic medullary osteo- sclerosis; case report, Bull. Hosp. Joint Dis. **15:**95, 1954.

77. Jansen, M.: Über atypische Chondrodys- trophie (Achondroplasie) und über eine noch nicht beschriebeni angeborene Wachstums- störung des Knochensystems: Metophysäre Dysostosis, Z. Orthop. Chir. **61:**253, 1934.

78. Bakwin, H., and Krida, A.: Familial meta- physial dysplasia, Amer. J. Dis. Child. **53:**1521, 1937.

79. Frank, W. W., and Denny, M. B.: Dysplasia epiphysealis punctata, J. Bone Joint Surg. **36-B:**118, 1954.

General reference

Fairbank, H. A. T.: An atlas of general affections of the skeleton, Edinburgh, 1951, E. & S. Liv- ingstone Ltd.

Chapter 3

Infections of bone

Pyogenic osteomyelitis

The widespread use of antibiotics has drastically altered the incidence and course of infection of bone by pyogenic organisms to the point where the pertinent articles of the 1920's and 1930's are now largely of historic interest.[1,2] One no longer has to stand by helplessly in the case of a child with acute hematogenous osteomyelitis while pus formed by *Staphylococcus aureus* or hemolytic streptococci spreads from the richly vascular metaphysis of a long bone up the medullary cavity and through the cortex to the periosteum. By the same token, today one seldom sees specimens of massive sequestrum resulting from thrombosis of nutrient vessels or of involucrum (a tube of cortical new bone deposited around a necrotic shaft as a core; Fig. 3-1). Also, the spread of infection to neighboring joints (pyarthrosis) with impairment of articular function, if not ankylosis, is no longer as serious a problem as it once was.[3] In many instances, the infection may be aborted, or at least significantly modified by adequate antibiotic therapy.

To be sure, chronic bone abscess is still very much a problem (Fig. 3-2), as is chronic osteomyelitis complicating compound fractures or orthopedic surgical procedures (a vexatious problem at times in hospital practice). Furthermore, antibiotic therapy has not altogether obviated the necessity for surgical drainage in cases of chronic osteomyelitis with small sequestra, pockets of residual infection, or persistent sinus tracts, for reasons to be indicated.

The pathologic reaction to infection in bone does not differ essentially from that in other tissues, although it is modified by the mineralized structure of bone in ways that can create special problems in successful treatment. As infected bone undergoes vascular and osteoclastic resorption, it is replaced by fibrous connective tissue. If the loss of bone is extensive, this can create a problem in reconstruction as well as in effective drainage. Also, as the periosteum is irritated, it lays down new cortical bone that can become quite dense (Fig. 3-3); this, too, may impede the evacuation of pus and sequestra. In these circumstances it is more difficult to attain adequate concentration of the antibiotic at the site of infection. Altogether, one can readily perceive why time-honored surgical procedures such as saucerization, removal of sequestra, and excision of sinus tracts must still be employed with some frequency to supplement the limited beneficial effect of antibiotic therapy, quite apart from the factor of bacterial resistance, through mutation, to specific antibiotic agents.

In *acute osteomyelitis* (as seen in a bone of a toe in a diabetic patient, for example), there are two cardinal histologic features: (1) extensive necrosis of bone, evidenced by loss of osteocytes in lacunae, and (2)

Fig. 3-1. Some bone specimens showing the changes in large limb bones of severe chronic osteomyelitis, as seen in the preantibiotic era. **A,** Large sequestrum in a tibia. **B,** Sequestrum in distal tibia with involucrum, and periosteal osteophytes on the contiguous fibula. **C,** Infection of the shaft of a femur with irregular periosteal new bone reaction. (From MacCallum, W. G.: A text-book of pathology, ed. 3, Philadelphia, 1924, W. B. Saunders Co.)

A   **B**

Fig. 3-2. A, Roentgenogram of a chronic bone abscess in the distal metaphysis of a radius. **B,** Another chronic bone abscess in the distal radius of an 8-year-old girl with a 2-year history.

Fig. 3-2, cont'd. **C**, Chronic bone abscess in the distal metaphysis of the humerus of a child. **D**, Cortical bone abscess in the distal femur of an adult. The possibility of a small osteoid-osteoma was also considered clinically.

Fig. 3-3. A, Roentgenogram showing a lesion of sclerosing osteomyelitis in the shaft of a metacarpal bone of an adult. Lesions such as this are sometimes referred to as the Garré type of osteomyelitis. **B,** Another instance of sclerosing osteomyelitis in the distal metaphysis of a radius, which simulated osteogenic sarcoma.

the presence of numerous pus cells (polymorphonuclear leukocytes) in the marrow spaces (Fig. 3-4, *A*). Similarly, in sections of an infected sequestrum one also finds dead bone and adherent pus or infected granulation tissue (Fig. 3-4, *B*).

In *chronic osteomyelitis,* there is more or less extensive resorption of bone and fibrous replacement. The residual bone may be rimmed by osteoblasts, reflecting an attempt at reconstruction. Within the fibrous tissue, there are numerous chronic inflammatory cells, including lymphocytes, plasma cells, and mononuclear macrophages; polymorphonuclear leukocytes are in a minority (Fig. 3-5, *A*). At times, these inflammatory cells may be so concentrated focally as to constitute a microabscess (Fig. 3-5, *B*).

In a *chronic bone abscess,* necrotic debris

and bacterial colonies may become walled off by fibrous tissue and inflamed granulation tissue (Fig. 3-6, *A*). Such an abscess may persist for years if it is not eradicated surgically, although culture may be sterile. Some surgeons are prone to designate any bone abscess as "Brodie's abscess," although Brodie in his old paper[*] actually described some five cases in point, *all in the tibia,* in which the manifestations of localized suppuration were ameliorated by drilling and evacuation of pus.

Because of their unusual effects, specific mention should be made in passing of osteomyelitis caused by certain bacteria other than the common pyogenic pathogens. *Salmonella* infection may be complicated oc-

---

[*]Available in reprints of the Sydenham Society.

Fig. 3-4. A, Photomicrograph of a focus of acute osteomyelitis showing necrosis of bone and the presence of pus in the marrow spaces. **B,** Infected sequestrum showing dead bone and adherent pus and infected granulation tissue.

casionally by bone abscess (Fig. 3-6, *B*) or by osteomyelitis in multiple foci, particularly in children and curiously in patients with sickle cell anemia. Unusual manifestations of osteomyelitis may also be caused by *B. proteus* and by *Klebsiella pneumoniae.*

In brucellosis, which is a particular problem in midwestern United States, bone and joint complications are well known, especially spondylitis (mainly at the lower thoracic and upper lumbar levels) with destruction of intervertebral disks and paravertebral abscess (simulating tuberculosis),

Fig. 3-5. A, Photomicrograph of a focus of chronic osteomyelitis. **B,** Another instance of chronic osteomyelitis, with a microabscess.

as well as osteomyelitis of long bones (with *Brucella suis* particularly). The antibiotic agents currently favored are the tetracycline derivatives and streptomycin used in combination, but these are not always as effective as they might be.

Attention should also be directed here to two possible sequelae of persistent chronic osteomyelitis of long standing, which are familiar to clinicians and pathologists alike: (1) amyloidosis, developing at times in patients with neglected or unsuccessfully treated infection, and (2) the appearance of malignant tumor in old sinus tracts, which may necessitate amputation. This is usually squamous cell carcinoma[4]

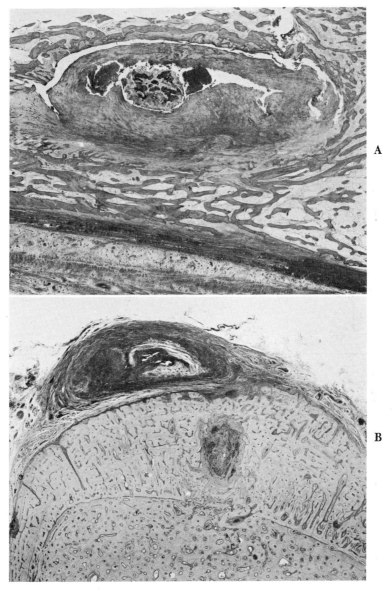

Fig. 3-6. A, Photomicrograph of a cortical chronic bone abscess of several years' standing. Although bacterial colonies were still discernible within this walled-off abscess, cultures were sterile. **B,** Periosteal abscess *(Salmonella)* overlying a layer of dense cortical new bone. The tract of infected granulation tissue within the thickened cortex was continuous at another level with the abscess on its surface. (This patient was found to have a sharply rising titer on Widal test, indicative of typhoid fever.)

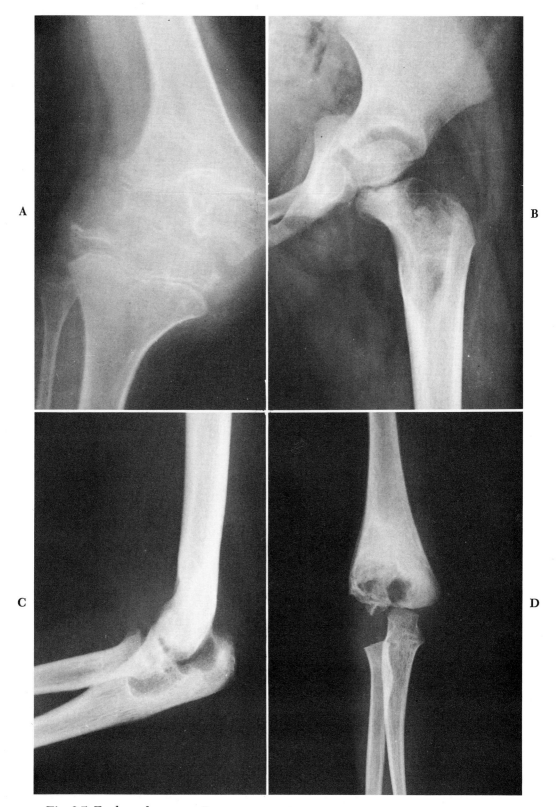

Fig. 3-7. For legend see opposite page.

E

F

G

Fig. 3-7. A, Roentgenogram of a young patient with tuberculosis of a knee, showing destructive changes in both articular bone ends, disuse atrophy, and some deformity. B, Tuberculosis of the upper metaphysis of the femur in a child. C, Tuberculosis of an elbow, involving the olecranon and the epicondyle of the humerus. D, Tuberculosis of the distal end of a humerus in a child 4 years of age. E, Tuberculous dactylitis of the middle phalanx of a fourth finger in a child. F, Tuberculosis of upper cervical spine, with retropharyngeal abscess. G, Tuberculosis of a first metatarsal bone in an adult who had earlier manifested skeletal tuberculosis elsewhere.

but, on rare occasions, it may be fibrosarcoma.[5] It seems altogether probable that these complications will occur with diminishing frequency in the future.

Skeletal tuberculosis

The advent of effective chemotherapy has had as great an impact on the incidence and course of bone and joint tuberculosis as it has on pyogenic osteomyelitis. Specifically, the widespread use of streptomycin and nicotinic acid hydrazides, especially iproniazid, has brought about a dramatic change, to the point that whole specialty hospitals formerly in great demand have gone out of business. Pott's disease with gibbus,[6-8] caries sicca (shoulder), and spina ventosa (tuberculous dactylitis) are just names to many younger medical men who see these conditions infrequently, if at all. For that matter, I now get most of my teaching material from Mexico, where skeletal tuberculosis is still prevalent (Fig. 3-7). For historic perspective, the reader may have profitable recourse to the authoritative account by Bosworth.[9]

To be sure, chemotherapy is not invariably successful and, as Bosworth indicates, the need for selected surgical procedures—particularly spine fusion for the stabilization of tuberculous spondylitis and arthrodesis of badly damaged weight-bearing joints—has not been entirely eliminated. But the surgeon can now do what he has to under specific antibiotic cover, without being fearful of local spread of infection, persistent sinus formation, or miliary dissemination.

The essential pathologic reaction to tuberculosis in skeletal structures is not essentially different from that in soft tissues. Productive (tubercle formation) and exudative aspects occur in varying proportion, depending largely upon the severity of the infection and the degree of acquired hypersensitivity of the patient. It may be remarked, however, that tubercles in bone are not likely to resemble the textbook picture, since they generally lack a mantle of lymphocytes and, frequently, Langhans' giant cells as well.

A few instances of serious bone infection simulating tuberculosis, caused by antibiotic resistant chromogenic acid-fast organisms (differing from *Mycobacterium tuberculosis* culturally and in other respects), have been cited by Aegerter and Kirkpatrick.[10] These authors also called attention to several cases of osteomyelitis caused by acid-fast organisms that provoked a tissue reaction resembling that of tuberculosis or leprosy, but that, because of their branching tendency on culture, were classified as *Nocardia*.

With further reference to infection by *Nocardia*, I had occasion to examine an amputated "Madura foot"[11] presenting numerous abscesses both in the bones and in the soft parts. In the vicinity of the abscesses there were branching colonies with clubs at their periphery, which morphologically resembled ray fungi but which were identified on culture as *Nocardia*.

Skeletal changes in leprosy

Leprosy, an ancient disease caused by *Mycobacterium leprae*, is not unknown in the United States.[12-14] There are endemic foci in Louisiana, for example; when I was at Charity Hospital in New Orleans, there were always a number of lepers there, as well as an appreciable number under treatment in the leprosarium at Carville.

This section will deal briefly with the skeletal alterations that may ensue in leprosy, especially in patients whose clinical manifestations have not been modified by prolonged sulfone therapy.

The most significant changes in the bones are associated with leprous neuritis or perineuritis (neural or anesthetic form). In this common expression of the disease, the scarring and cord-like thickening of nerve bundles lead to loss of sensation, striking trophic changes in the extremities, and eventual mutilation of the hands and feet, with claw-like contractures or hideous stumps that may develop penetrating ulcers. It appears that secondary infection is a contributing factor in this process. In the cutaneous form of leprosy, there may be secondary destruction of the cartilage of the nose and even of the bones of the face. Finally, there is also a kind of leprous osteomyelitis as part of advanced systemic dissemination, with lesions analogous to those of the skin, but this is much less significant than the sequelae of neural involvement.

The pathologic reaction is featured by foamy macrophages (lepra cells) and sometimes by giant cells as well. Acid-fast bacilli are found not only in these cells but also in large numbers in endothelial cells of the granulation tissue. In the interpretation of skin biopsies particularly, the diagnosis of leprosy can be overlooked by an unwary observer through failure to do an acid-fast stain.

Skeletal involvement in granuloma inguinale

Granuloma inguinale, long held to be a venereal disease affecting young adults of both sexes, especially Negroes, is quite familiar to physicians who have worked in the southern part of the United States. The condition characteristically involves the genital region (including the cervix in women) and/or the inguinal region. Only infrequently does it affect extragenital sites as well. The infection is apparently caused by Donovan bodies, which appear as intracellular inclusions and which are best demonstrated by Giemsa or Wright's stain. Dissemination, presumably hematogenous, does occur occasionally, so that a few instances of skeletal involvement have been reported.[15-17] In one such instance,[15] for example, there was osteomyelitis of the spine that destroyed the fourth lumbar vertebra and part of the fifth. Giemsa stain of a needle aspiration biopsy showed intracellular Donovan bodies in large number. It is noteworthy that the condition was successfully treated by chloramphenicol and subsequent spine fusion.

Skeletal manifestations of syphilis

Although the control of syphilis, a common venereal disease, is still a serious public health problem, the availability of penicillin has dramatically reduced the incidence of its skeletal complications. Specifically, the use of penicillin in prenatal clinics has made the osseous manifestations of congenital lues far less common than they used to be, while gummatous syphilis in the adult is now seldom observed in hospital practice. For detailed accounts of the former skeletal ravages of syphilis one must have recourse to old texts and articles[13,18-21] or, by analogy, to current descriptions of the effects of *yaws* (a related, penicillin-sensitive, spirochetal infection), as seen in Africa and the South Pacific, for example. The superbly illustrated monograph of Hackett[22] on the bone lesions of yaws in Uganda is particularly recommended.

The best known and most consistent manifestation of untreated or inadequately treated *congenital syphilis* is osteochondritis of the upper and lower limb bones, which often leads to epiphyseal separation (Fig. 3-8, *A*). The spirochetes fluorish in the richly vascular growth zones, and their noxious effect and the resulting inflammatory exudate disrupt the process of endochondral ossification (Fig. 3-8, *B*). Irregularity and widening of the affected zone are reflected roentgenographically, and a yellow line is grossly discernible.

Periostitis or osteoperiostitis affecting the shaft of the long bones, especially those of the leg, forearm, and hand, is another relatively frequent manifestation in infancy and is found occasionally in older children. Gummas may form in affected bones (as they may elsewhere), particularly in long bones or the skull, and the gummatous nodes can undergo softening and suppuration with sinus formation.

Severe untreated infection results in death of the fetus or neonate. Those who survive may go on to show such familiar late manifestations as interstitial keratitis; deformed teeth, particularly the upper central incisors of the second set (Hutchinson's teeth); leukoderma; nerve deafness; juvenile taboparesis; saddle nose (from destruction of the septum and turbinates); saber shin (from osteoperiostitis of the tibia); dactylitis, with spindle-shaped enlargement[18,22]; and occasionally chronic synovitis, especially of knee joints (Clutton's joints).[23]

The skeletal changes of *acquired syphilis* include periostitis, resulting in irregularly dense bony thickening (hyperostosis), and formation of gummas, especially in the calvarium and long bones (Fig. 3-8, C). Specific joint involvement (synovitis of large joints, especially the knee, with effusion) once seen as an occasional manifestation has become a rarity, although damage to articular cartilage may result from involvement of contiguous bone ends. To be sure, more or less extensive destruction of weight-bearing joints secondary to tabes (Charcot's joint), especially in the lower extremity and the vertebral column, is still a formidable clinical problem. This will be discussed further on in the section on neurotrophic disorders of joints (see Chapter 9).

Bone involvement in fungus infections—coccidiomycosis

Of all the fungus infections that may be manifested in osseous lesions coccidiomycosis is by far the most common, at least in the Central Valley of California, in southwestern United States, and in the adjacent arid states of northern Mexico (fungi do not respect geographic boundaries). By comparison, skeletal lesions in other pathogenic mycoses—such as actinomycosis, blastomycosis, histoplasmosis, cryptococcosis,

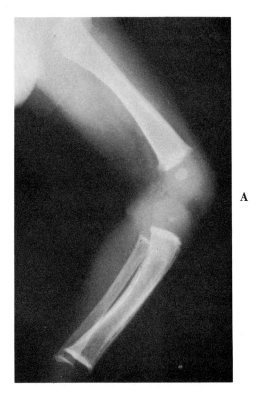

A

Fig. 3-8. **A**, Roentgenogram showing the changes of osteochondritis in congenital syphilis. **B**, Photomicrograph showing luetic osteochondritis of the distal femur in a dead neonate examined at autopsy. (The mother had received only partial, inadequate treatment in prenatal clinic.) Note disruption of endochondral ossification at the plate. Special stain showed spirochetes in abundance within the inflammatory exudate. **C**, Photomicrograph of a partially necrotic, destructive skeletal focus (one of many) in a South Pacific native with yaws. The area of necrosis is bordered by inflamed granulation tissue containing occasional histiocytic nodes. This picture is quite analogous to that of gummatous syphilis.

and sporotrichosis—are unusual, if not rare.

Although coccidiomycosis is primarily and predominantly a self-limited pulmonary disease, as Forbus[24] and others have pointed out, the bones (and occasionally the joints as well) are among the more

Fig. 3-8, cont'd. For legend see opposite page.

common sites of infection resulting from hematogenous dissemination of *Coccidioides immitis*.[25,26] One or more osseous sites may be affected. There is a curious predilection for bony prominences such as the radial styloid, tibial tubercle, malleoli of the ankle, olecranon, acromion, and sternoclavicular area, although the skull, vertebral column, ribs, and sternum, as well as other bones, may also be involved on occasion. Infection at any of these sites may be complicated by suppuration and persistent sinus formation. Incidentally, there is a widely held belief that skeletal involvement in dissemination is inevitably serious, but there are undoubtedly cases in which

51

Fig. 3-9. A, Roentgenogram showing a lesion of coccidiomycosis in the distal radius and adjacent soft parts (sinus formation). The patient was a Filipino male adult who had had exacerbations from time to time over a period of almost 10 years. **B,** Coccidiomycosis causing collapse of a cervical vertebra (in a young adult Negro). Diagnosis was established by needle aspiration (see Fig. 3-10).

the clinical course is chronic and protracted over a period of many years (Fig. 3-9, *A*). No altogether satisfactory chemotherapeutic agent has as yet been discovered for coccidiomycosis, although a number have been given clinical trial over the years, and the search continues.

The pathologic response to *Coccidioides immitis* has both suppurative and granulomatous aspects, and frequently the two are combined (Fig. 3-10). When healing occurs in lesions that have gone beyond early resolution, it is usually a result of scarring and hyalinization (as may occur in tuberculosis). In predominantly granulomatous lesions, the mimicry of the tuberculous reaction may be remarkable; it is only by meticulous search for the spherules

of *Coccidioides immitis* (often found within giant cells) that the problem in differentiation can be readily resolved.

Unusual expressions of mycotic osteomyelitis. In *actinomycosis,* involvement of bones (as well as of joints and paraskeletal connective tissues) usually results from direct extension and burrowing of neighboring soft tissue lesions. Specifically, this may move from the mouth to the mandible (analogous to "lumpy jaw" of cattle); from the lungs to the ribs and even vertebrae; from the ileocecal region to the lumbar spine, sacrum, or iliac bone; or from the skin, burrowing into deeper tissues, including fascia, bones, and joints.[27-29]

That the ray fungus may cause infection in man has been known since 1879.[30] A

C

good account of its pathologic manifestations may be found in MacCallum.[13] In essence, the tissue reaction, wherever it may be, is characterized by destruction and liquefaction, with abscess and sinus formation. The branched organisms grow in tangled mycelia (strahlenpilz), and colonies found in pus may appear as yellow "sulfur" granules. In tissue sections, one may have to make an extended search through many levels to find a single ray fungus, which suffices for a firm diagnosis.

Although osteomyelitis caused by the fungus *Blastomyces dermatitidis* was described as early as 1894 by Gilchrist, this manifestation is infrequent in man.[31,32] Infection of bone may develop by deep extension of cutaneous lesions (for example,

Fig. 3-9, cont'd. C, Roentgenograms of a destructive focus in the distal metaphysis of the radius of a child, which proved on tissue examination to be a lesion of coccidiomycosis.

Fig. 3-10. Photomicrograph of a needle aspiration biopsy of the lesion shown in Fig. 3-9, B. The response in this instance was an acute inflammatory one, but the presence of scattered spherules of *Coccidioides immitis* confirmed the diagnosis.

on an extremity) or, more often, from hematogenous dissemination with systemic involvement. In the latter circumstance, destructive lesions may develop in the vertebral column, in limb bones, or elsewhere. Such lesions have been described radiographically as simulating skeletal tuberculosis rather than pyogenic osteomyelitis.

Diagnosis is established by the finding in pus or in tissue specimens of doubly refractile blastomyces, which tend to be engulfed by foreign body giant cells. With reference to therapy, aromatic diamidines have been found effective against systemic blastomycosis (and possibly other systemic fungus infections).[33]

Sporotrichosis, caused by a filamentous spore-forming fungus (*Sporotrichium*), produces bone lesions only rarely in man.[34] Although these were recorded as early as 1898 by Shenk, I have never observed a case of this disease. As in some other fungus infections, osteomyelitis is described as developing either by direct selection from an overlying ulcer or abscess or by hematogenous spread. In the latter event, the skeletal lesions may be multiple,[35] affecting the skull, ribs, long bones, and phalanges (simulating the dactylitis of syphilis or tuberculosis).

Cryptococcosis (torulosis) and *histoplasmosis,* while relatively common fungus infections,[36] only infrequently produce clinically detectable bone lesions.[37-40] However, infection of the knee joint (pyarthrosis) has been reported in both conditions.[41] Curiously enough, in each instance the condition was thought to be tuberculous arthritis until the causative organisms were identified.

Lesions of bone caused by parasitic disease

Of all the numerous diseases in man caused by animal parasites, only one is relevant here, that caused by the cestode worm *Taenia echinococcus,* for which man may be the intermediate host (the mature form is a parasite of the intestine of the dog). The disease is most common in sheep raising areas;[42] it is seen only occasionally in the United States. The parasitic eggs are transmitted to the human digestive tract, and the wandering of the embryos can take them to any organ of the body, where they develop as huge cysts (or hydatids) with daughter cysts and scolices contained by chitinous walls. Localization in bone and the development of significant disease there are said to occur in no more than 1% of the cases of infestation with recognized clinical disease.

As a rule, only a single bone is affected by echinococcosis. Its site, of course, is fortuitous,[42-45] although involvement of the vertebral column, especially of the thoracic spine, appears to be relatively frequent.[7] The disease may remain localized, or it may slowly extend to involve the entire bone. Radiographically such lesions are described as "cystic and multilocular," with little or no expansion of the cortex and no periosteal new bone reaction. Pathologic fracture may occur, with some hazard of spread.

The only effective treatment is complete surgical excision, although this may not always be feasible.

Bone changes in viral infections

The finding of osseous lesions in *smallpox* is an old observation.[46,47] In children, growth arrest and premature fusion of epiphyses have been described. It appears also that in adults, as well as in children, nonsuppurative osteomyelitis (designated "osteomyelitis variolosa" in older literature[48]) may be a sequel of smallpox, as may also arthritis of the elbow and other joints, ending in ankylosis and deformity. That these skeletal complications are not rare is evidenced by the fact that Bose[49] reported as many as twelve cases from Calcutta, where smallpox is still prevalent. He could not be certain whether the osteoarticular lesions resulted from the viral lesion per se or whether some of them may not have reflected secondary pyogenic infection in debilitated young patients.

In *rubella* (German measles), bone changes in the newborn held to be specific and "virtually diagnostic" have been reported by Singleton and his associates at Texas Children's Hospital in Houston. These infants were born of mothers who had had rubella during the first trimester of pregnancy (contracted during the course of an epidemic); they showed, in addition to the usual defects of cataracts and cardiac anomalies, thrombocytopenic purpura, a large anterior fontanelle, and, on roentgenographic survey, poorly defined irregular growth plates and altered trabecular patterns in the metaphyses of long bones, especially of the distal femora and proximal tibiae.

Aegerter and Kirkpatrick[10] have briefly cited an instance in which "multiple areas

of bone destruction" appeared in a patient with severe *vaccinia* (the patient eventually recovered).

Osteolytic lesions have also been described as complications in occasional patients with *cat-scratch fever*,[50] although their precise nature was not clearly stated. Bone and joint infections of pyogenic nature have also been noted as unusual complications of *chickenpox*.[51]

Infantile cortical hyperostosis (*Caffey's disease*)

Infantile cortical hyperostosis, first delineated by Caffey and Silverman[52] in 1945, affects young infants, particularly between 2 and 6 months of age. It is characterized pathologically by a peculiar inflammatory osteoperiostitis found most often in the long limb bones, mandible, clavicles, ribs, and scapulae. Occasionally other bones may be affected as well. The condition is

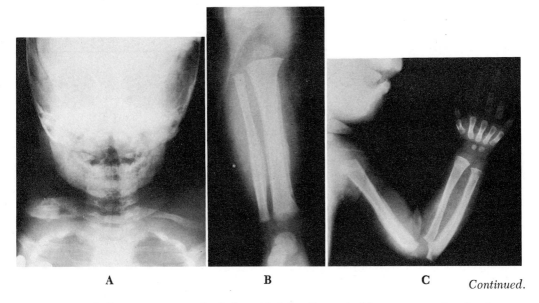

A   B   C   *Continued.*

Fig. 3-11. **A,** Roentgenogram of a baby with infantile cortical hyperostoses showing involvement of the mandible bilaterally and of a clavicle. The long limb bones were not examined. **B,** Periosteal new bone apposition on the tibia and fibula of another infant with Caffey's disease. **C,** Comparable changes in the humerus and ulna. Note also the enlargement of the lower jaw.

Fig. 3-11, cont'd. **D**, Low power photomicrograph of a cross section of an affected bone in infantile cortical hyperostosis. **E**, Photomicrograph at higher magnification showing the character of the granulation tissue within the thickened cortex of the bone illustrated in **D**.

by no means uncommon and is being recognized with increasing frequency in pediatric practice[53-56] (Fig. 3-11, *A*, *B*, and *C*).

Clinically, infantile cortical hyperostosis is commonly ushered in by fever, irritability, and tender indurated swellings at sites where bone lesions appear. During the acute phase, anemia, leukocytosis, elevated sedimentation rate, and pleural thickening and exudate may also be present. The condition is usually self-limited, although I have had an unusual opportunity to examine the bones in an autopsied case of a baby who developed thrombocytopenia and fatal cerebral hemorrhage (Fig. 3-11, *D* and *E*). There may be periods of remission and exacerbation, but, as a rule, the manifestations subside after some weeks or months, and the affected bones undergo gradual reconstruction that is said to be substantially complete by 3 years of age.[57] Only rarely, apparently, do bowing deformities persist beyond early childhood.[56]

Radiographically, in the active phase of the disease the affected bones characteristically show more or less prominent periosteal new bone apposition (Fig. 3-11). This bone apposition may be lamellated and extensive and may lead to club-like thickening and deformity of the long limb bones (hyperostoses). These changes, although distinctive, may initially suggest scurvy, luetic osteoperiostitis, or severe trauma. As indicated, the cortical thickening gradually diminishes and tends to disappear after several months.

The essential pathologic lesion in affected bones, at least in the active stage of the disease, is a peculiar inflammatory osteoperiostitis (Fig. 3-11, *D* and *E*). As noted in Fig. 3-11, *D*, a photomicrograph of a cross section of a thickened affected bone (one of many examined at autopsy), there is partial resorption of the original cortex and, layered over it, concentric tiers of cortical new bone, the trabeculae of which are oriented, for the most part, at right angles to the attenuated original cortex. Fig. 3-11, *E*, at higher magnification, shows the nature of the granulation tissue within the thickened cortex. In addition to numerous fibroblasts, there are large histiocytes and an inflammatory exudate featuring small mononuclear cells and only an occasional polymorphonuclear leukocyte. In the matter of interpretation, as I see it, this type of reaction is quite consistent with the concept of a viral infection.

Caffey[52] suggests that infantile cortical hyperostosis might well be an infection, possibly viral in nature. This working hypothesis would indeed explain many of the clinical features of this disease, particularly the fever, leukocytosis, elevated sedimentation rate, and pleurisy with mononuclear exudate, as well as the peculiar inflammatory osteoperiostitis observed pathologically in the affected bones. It has also been suggested that there may be a hereditary or familial factor, based on occasional reports of incidence in two or three members of a family and, more importantly, on an account of eleven cases in a single family over a 14-year period.[53,56] While the latter observation is noteworthy, the familial incidence cited may reflect opportunity for contagion rather than a hereditary congenital disorder. It is conceivable also that adults can harbor a virus for a long time (as with herpes simplex) and transmit it to susceptible young infants in the kindred. Altogether, it appears to me that one should reserve judgment concerning this problem of etiology, pending further study.

References

1. Wilensky, A. O.: Osteomyelitis, New York, 1934, The Macmillan Co.
2. Wilson, J. C., and McKeever, F. M.: Hematogenous acute osteomyelitis in children, J. Bone Joint Surg. 18:323, 1936.
3. Steindler, A.: Pyogenic arthritis: the musculoskeletal system: a symposium, New York, 1952, The Macmillan Co., pp. 287-312.
4. Sedlin, E. D., and Fleming, J. L.: Epidermoid

carcinoma arising in chronic osteomyelitic foci, J. Bone Joint Surg. **45-A**:827-838, 1963.

5. Morris, J. M., and Lucas, D. B.: Fibrosarcoma within a sinus tract of chronic draining osteomyelitis, J. Bone. Joint Surg. **46-A**:853, 1964.

6. Carr, E. F.: Tuberculosis of the spine in children, Clin. Orthop., No. 1, p. 129.

7. Schmorl, G., and Junghanns, H.: Die Gesunde und die Kranke Wirbelsäüle in Roentgenbild und Klinik, ed. 4, Stuttgart, 1957, Georg Thieme Verlag.

8. Sanchis Olmos, V.: La tuberculosis del esqueleto, Barcelona, 1957, Editorial Ciéntifico Medica.

9. Bosworth, D. M.: Treatment of tuberculosis of bone and joint, Bull. N. Y. Acad. Med. **35**:167-177, 1959.

10. Aegerter, E., and Kirkpatrick, J. A., Jr.: Orthopedic diseases, ed. 2, Philadelphia, 1963, W. B. Saunders Co., pp. 263-265.

11. Oyston, J. K.: Madura foot, a study of twenty cases, J. Bone Joint Surg. **43-B**: 259, 1961.

12. Harbitz: Arch. Intern. Med. **6**:147, 1910.

13. McCallum, W. G.: A text-book of pathology, ed. 3, Philadelphia, 1924, W. B. Saunders Co.

14. Veterans Administration Technical Bulletin: Leprosy, TB 10-98, Washington, D. C., March 15, 1954. (For literature on treatment, particularly.)

15. Kalstone, B. M., Howell, J. A., Jr., and Cline, F. X., Jr.: Granuloma inguinale with hematogenous dissemination to the spine, J.A.M.A. **176**:152, 1961.

16. Lyford, J., III, Scott, R. B., and Johnson, R. W., Jr.: Polyarticular arthritis and osteomyelitis due to granuloma inguinale, Amer. J. Syph. **28**:588, 1944.

17. Rajam, R. V., Rangiati, P. N., and Anguli, V. C.: Systemic donovaniasis, Brit. J. Vener. Dis. **30**:73, 1954.

18. Hodges, P. C., Phemister, D. E., and Brunschwig, A.: The roentgen-ray diagnosis of diseases of the bones and joints, New York, 1938, Thomas Nelson and Sons, pp. 37-48.

19. Holt, L. E., and Howland, J.: Diseases of infancy and childhood, ed. 9, New York, 1926, D. Appleton and Co., pp. 917-944.

20. Freund, E.: Über Knochensyphilis, Virch. Arch. Path. Anat. **288**:146, 1933.

21. Pick, L.: Angeborene Knochensyphilis. In Henke and Lubarsch: Handbuch. der spec. Anatomie und Histologie, Berlin, 1929, Springer Verlag, p. 240.

22. Hackett, C. J.: Bone lesions of yaws in Uganda, Oxford, 1951, Blackwell Scientific Publications.

23. Argen, R. J., and Dixon, A. St. J.: Clutton's joints with keratitis and periostitis: a case report with histology of synovium, Arthritis Rheum. **6**:341-348, 1963.

24. Forbus, W. D., and Bestebreurtje, A. M.: Coccidiomycosis: a study of 95 cases of the disseminated type with special reference to the pathogenesis of the disease, Mil. Surg. **99**:653-719, 1946. (Well-documented references through 1945.)

25. Carter, R. A.: Infectious granulomas of bones and joints, with special reference to coccidioidal granuloma, Radiology **23**:1-16, 1934.

26. McMaster, P. E., and Gilfillan, C. F.: Coccidioidal osteomyelitis, J.A.M.A. **112**:1233-1237, 1939.

27. Parker, C. A.: Actinomycosis and blastomycosis of spine, J. Bone Joint Surg. **5**:759, 1923.

28. Rhangos, W. C., and Chick, E. W.: Mycotic infections of bone, Southern Med. J. **57**:664-674, 1964.

29. Simpson, W. M., and McIntosh, C. A.: Actinomycosis of vertebrae (actinomycotic Pott's disease); report of 4 cases, Arch. Surg. **14**: 116, 1927.

30. Israel: Virch. Arch. **74**:15, 1879; ibid. **78**:421, 1879.

31. Colonna, P. A., and Gucker, T.: Blastomycosis of the skeletal system, J. Bone Joint Surg. **26**:322, 1944.

32. Martin, D. S., and Smith, D. T.: Blastomycosis (review of literature), Amer. Rev. Tuberc. **39**:275, 488, 1938.

33. Editorial: Diamidine therapy of blastomycosis, J.A.M.A. **154**:588, 1954.

34. Foerster, H. R.: Sporotrichosis, Amer. J. Med. Sci. **167**:54, 1924.

35. Reeves, R. J., and Pedersen, R.: Fungus infection of bone, Radiology **62**:55, 1954.

36. Mitchel, L. A.: Torulosis, J.A.M.A. **106**:450, 1936.

37. Allcock, E. A.: Torulosis, J. Bone Joint Surg. **43-B**:71, 1961.

38. Allen, J. H.: Bone involvement with disseminated histoplasmosis, Amer. J. Roentgen. **82**:250, 1959.

39. Durie, E. B., and MacDonald, L.: Cryptococcosis (torulosis) of bone, report of a case, J. Bone Joint Surg. **43-B**:68, 1961.

40. Klingberg, W. G.: Generalized histoplasmosis in infants and children: review of 10 cases with apparent recovery: J. Pediat. **36**:728, 1950.

41. Key, J. A., and Large, H. M.: Histoplasmosis of the knee, J. Bone Joint Surg. **24**:28, 1942.

42. Dew, H. R.: Hydatid disease: its pathology, diagnosis, and treatment, Sydney, 1928, Australasian Medical Publishing Co.

43. Coley, B. L.: Echinococcus disease of bone;

report of 2 cases involving pelvic girdle, J. Bone Joint Surg. **14:**577, 1932.

44. Howorth, M. B.: Echinococcus of bone (includes review of literature), J. Bone Joint Surg. **27:**401, 1945.

45. Hsieh, C. K.: Echinococcus involvement of bone; report of case, Radiology **14:**562, 1930.

46. Chiari, H.: Beitr. Path. Anat. **13:**13, 1893.

47. Musgrave, W. E., and Sison, A. G.: Bone lesions of smallpox, Philippine J. Sci. **5:**553, 1910; ibid. **8:**67, 1913.

48. Brown, W. L., and Brown, C. P.: Osteomyelitis variolosa, J.A.M.A. **81:**1414, 1923.

49. Bose, K. S.: Osteo-articular lesions in smallpox, J. Indian Med. Ass. **31:**151, 1958.

50. Carithers, H. A., Carithers, C. M., and Edwards, R. O., Jr.: Cat-scratch disease: its natural history, J.A.M.A. **207:**312, 1969.

51. Buck, R. E.: Pyarthrosis of the hip complicating chickenpox, J.A.M.A. **206:**136, 1968.

52. Caffey, J., and Silverman, W. A.: Infantile cortical hyperostoses: preliminary report on a new syndrome, Amer. J. Roentgen. **54:**1-16, 1945.

53. Editorial: Caffey's enigma, J.A.M.A. **175:**495, 1961.

54. Sherman, M. S., and Hillyer, D. T.: Infantile cortical hyperostosis: review of literature and report of five cases, Amer. J. Roentgen. **63:**212, 1950.

55. Smyth, F. S., Potter, A., and Silverman, W.: Periosteal reaction, fever and irritability in young infants: new syndrome, Amer. J. Dis. Child. **71:**333-350, 1946.

56. Tampas, J. P., van Buskirk, F. W., Peterson, O. S., and Soule, A. B.: Infantile cortical hyperostosis, J.A.M.A. **175:**167, 1961.

57. Caffey, J.: On some late skeletal changes in chronic infantile cortical hyperostosis, Radiology **59:**651, 1952.

Chapter 4

Skeletal changes in vitamin deficiencies and excesses

This chapter is concerned primarily with vitamin C deficiency (scurvy) and vitamin D deficiency (rickets and osteomalacia), and to a lesser extent with vitamin A deficiency. As for excessive administration, only the effects of vitamins A and D are relevant; inordinately large amounts of vitamin C (ascorbic acid) are apparently not harmful.

Vitamin A deficiency

There is an optimal range of vitamin A dosage, just as there is for other dietary essentials; deviations in either direction have been demonstrated to have deleterious effects. Vitamin A deficiency in infants was recognized[1] as early as 1933, but the condition is uncommon and only a limited number of case reports[2-5] has appeared since then. If the diet of the pregnant mother is extremely low in vitamin A, or if she is suffering from a malabsorption syndrome, the newborn infant may have low stores of vitamin A or even clinical vitamin A deficiency.[5,6]

The most consistent manifestation of such a deficiency is xerophthalmia (keratitis and scarring of the cornea, with impairment of vision) but many other signs have been noted,[7,8] among them mental and physical retardation, cornification of

vaginal epithelium, refractory anemia, and some rather curious neurologic changes such as facial palsy, seventh cranial nerve injury, and hydrocephalus. The skeletal alterations are not particularly noteworthy and relate to the general impairment of growth and development.[4] There may also be defective enamel and dentin formation in developing teeth.

Vitamin A excess or poisoning
(hypervitaminosis A)

The harmful effects of hypervitaminosis A in infants and young children were described[9] in 1944. Subsequently, an appreciable number of similar reports appeared in the pediatric and radiologic literature.[10,11]

Hypervitaminosis A is characterized by anorexia, loss of weight, irritability, pruriginous rash, sparseness of hair, and hepatomegaly, as well as by swelling, pain, and tenderness over affected bones. The latter are usually long limb bones, although other bones such as the foot bones and calvarium may be involved. On roentgenographic examination, they show periosteal new bone apposition, the appearance of which is not unlike that of the milder expressions of infantile cortical hyperostosis (Fig. 4-1).

The clinical histories of such babies and

Fig. 4-1. **A,** Roentgenogram of a 2-year-old child with hypervitaminosis A showing cortical thickening from periosteal new bone apposition on the shaft of a femur. **B,** Comparable changes in the shaft of an ulna in the same case.

young children indicate, as a rule, entirely too much vitamin A in their diets, often supplemented by excessive amounts of vitamin A concentrate administered in error or through ignorance of its consequences. The suggestion has been advanced[11] that inability of the liver to store and handle the vitamin (hepatic dysfunction) is a contributing factor. Be that as it may, the toxic manifestations soon disappear when the condition is corrected, although the bone changes persist for some time, as one might expect.

There are some relevant experimental data that should be mentioned here. As Cohlan[12] has pointed out, the administration of excessive amounts of vitamin A to pregnant rats produces a diminished litter rate[13,14] and characteristic congenital malformations among the surviving young,

commonly defective calvarium with extrusion of the brain, and, sporadically, other anomalies such as macroglossia, harelip, cleft palate, and gross defects in eye development. Another interesting observation[15] is that, in rabbits, cartilage can be dissolved by excess vitamin A; however, this effect can be prevented by the administration of cortisone.

Vitamin C deficiency—scurvy
(scorbutus; Möller-Barlow's disease; avitaminosis C)

Because of its obvious and dramatic features, scurvy, especially in sailors and professional soldiers, has been known for a long time.[16] In fact, the word came into colloquial use as an adjective, in the sense of mean or contemptible (such as a scurvy trick). However, the delineation of this

61

Fig. 4-2. A, Sagittal section of the femur of a young child who died of scurvy. (From MacCallum, W. G.: A text-book of pathology, ed. 3, Philadelphia, 1924, W. B. Saunders Co.) **B,** Roentgenogram showing changes in the growth zones of both femora and tibiae in infantile scurvy, as well as striking periosteal new bone formation in consequence of subperiosteal hemorrhage.

deficiency disease in clinical and pathologic terms proceeded at a pedestrian pace.

Although the curative effect of lemon (and lime) juice was discovered as early as 1753 by Lind,[16] it took more than a century thereafter for infantile scurvy to be clearly established as a clinical entity distinct from rickets and other disorders,[17] and another 25 years for scurvy to be produced experimentally in guinea pigs.[18] The elucidation of its pathologic changes came even later, while the classical chemical analysis and identification of vitamin C as ascorbic acid by Szent-Györgi dates back to 1928.

As is now well known, full-blown clinical scurvy is characterized by progressive secondary anemia, weakness, slight fever, swelling, bleeding and ulceration of the gums (with loosening of teeth), exquisite tenderness of the legs from painful hemorrhages about the joints and under the periosteum (particularly of long limb bones), and ecchymoses in the skin, muscles, and internal organs (kidney and bowel). The condition may be fatal if left untreated, since infections, especially pneumonia, may develop. On the other hand, rapid healing occurs following vitamin C administration, although it may be several months before

Fig. 4-2, cont'd. C, Photomicrograph of a growth plate in severe infantile scurvy showing disruption of endochondral ossification. The columns of calcified cartilage are broken up and enmeshed in an irregular zone of necrosis and hemorrhage.

there is complete restoration of the skeletal structures.

Scurvy is now unusual in adults except under war starvation conditions, but it may be seen occasionally in alcoholics, extreme diet faddists, or the very deprived. It is still observed in young children (usually from 6 to 15 months of age) who are fed boiled or condensed milk and no citrus juices. Subclinical vitamin C deficiency is believed to be not uncommon and is a possible cause of delayed wound healing.[19]

Pathologically, if one examines a long limb bone of a young scorbutic subject (Fig. 4-2, A), two unusual features are immediately apparent:

1. Hemorrhages may be found within the bone marrow (most conspicuous at the growing end of the bone) and also under the periosteum, which may be elevated over a large part of the shaft by the effusion of blood and which tends to form reactive new bone.[20,21] This is, of course, reflected roentgenographically and the changes may be quite striking (Fig. 4-2, B).

2. The growth zone is broadened and irregular, reflecting stagnation or cessation of bone formation through endochondral ossification. More specifically, there is lack of orderly invasion of calcified cartilage columns by osteoblastic vascular connective tissue, so that only sparse, scattered trabeculae of new bone are formed, or none at all.

An adequate concentration of vitamin C is required for the formation of collagen and ground substance,[22] which constitute the substratum of osteoid and bone. In severe lesions there is complete disruption of this portion of the plate, with necrosis and hemorrhage (Fig. 4-2, C). Epiphyseal separation may occur and is often bilateral.

This is observed most often in the lower femur, upper tibia, and upper humerus. There may also be costochondral separations.

Further, as a consequence of stagnation of new bone formation, whereas resorption proceeds normally (and is, in fact, accelerated by disuse or immobilization), there is a tendency to thinning of cortices and atrophy of the spongiosa, reflected roentgenographically in a washed-out appearance. As for the marrow, this in time loses its myeloid elements as well as its blood vessels and osteoblasts and is converted to an edematous fibrous tissue. It is remarkable that these profound changes are reversible, as noted, if vitamin C therapy is not too long delayed.

Vitamin D deficiency

Rickets. At one time, rickets was probably, at least in northern cities, the disease from which infants most frequently suffered. In fact, among the poor in these cities it was an almost universal disease.[23] As the administration of vitamin D in one form or another to babies became routine pediatric practice,[24-27] the incidence of rickets, at least in severe form, declined sharply, to the point that pathologic teaching material is now hard to come by. To be sure, it was recognized some 40 years ago that ultraviolet light and/or potent fish liver oils could heal rickets; what has happened is that we have moved ahead from good treatment to effective prevention. That is not to say that rickets may not still be encountered at times, particularly in its mild or subclinical expressions, or even in its advanced stage under unusual circumstances.[28]

Rickets is one of the so-called malacic diseases of bone. Its most striking feature is the presence of osteoid (limeless bone) throughout the skeleton. As a result of vitamin D deficiency the osteoid is not calcified and converted to bone. It has been cogently postulated that in the absence of

Fig. 4-3. A, Sections through the bones of a 14-month-old baby showing the changes of active rickets (the cause of death was bronchopneumonia). **B,** Conspicuous enlargement of costochondral junctions in the same child.

adequate vitamin D there is faulty absorption of calcium from the gut (such intestinal disorders as idiopathic steatorrhea, celiac disease, or sprue may sometimes be a contributing factor); that the parathyroid homeostatic mechanism acts to maintain the serum calcium level by drawing calcium out of the skeleton; and that parathyroid hyperactivity concomitantly brings about the loss of phosphorus through the kidneys. Thus the serum phosphorus level is consistently low in rickets (as low as 1.0 mg./100 ml. in extreme cases), while the serum calcium level is likely to be in the low normal range. The stimulus to new bone formation by way of attempted reconstruction is reflected in significantly elevated alkaline phosphatase activity in the serum. The latter returns to normal only slowly and may remain somewhat increased even after clinical and roentgenographic evidence of healing is manifest.

When rickets is observed clinically, it begins usually at 6 to 18 months of age and lasts for several to many months, sometimes for years, with remissions and final healing. The active process ends, as a rule, by the time the child is 2 or 2½ years old in all but the severe or resistant cases. The disease has systemic effects and, at the height of its development, the old commonplace picture was that of a pale, sickly child restless at night and sweating about the head, with secondary anemia, lowered resistance to infection, lymphadenopathy (especially of tonsils, adenoids, and cervical nodes), protrusion of the abdomen (potbelly), splenomegaly (from hyperplasia), retarded dentition, poor development and flabbiness of musculature, and laxity of ligaments. The most constant and characteristic lesions, however, are found in the skeleton. There is enlargement of epiphyses (especially at the wrists, knees, and ankles) and of costochondral junctions (beaded ribs or rachitic rosary). There may also be thoracic deformity, scoliosis,

bending or greenstick fractures of long bones (particularly of the forearm bones and femora), deformed pelvis, bowing of femora and tibiae (knock knees), and coxa vara from general softening and thinning of the bones. There is also enlargement of the skull with prominent forehead (spongy thickenings over the frontal and parietal fossas) and thin occiput (craniotabes). The capacity for skeletal reconstruction in young children is so remarkable, fortunately, that most cases end with gradual restoration of normal consistency and structure of affected bones. If orthopedic corrective measures are neglected, however, the changes described may leave lasting deformities in adults, notably of the chest (with diminished vital capacity) and of the pelvis (with narrowed outlet, interfering with parturition in women), as well as flat feet, coxa vara, scoliosis, and the familiar bowlegs and knock knees.

The changes outlined are, of course, reflected roentgenographically and are of diagnostic importance, as are also the altered serum chemistry findings. In essence, the significant roentgenographic alterations relate to failure of centers of ossification in epiphyses to appear or to be clearly outlined (osteoid is not radiopaque); to demineralization of the skeleton (in variable degree and for the reason previously indicated); and, most importantly, to irregular broadening of epiphyseal cartilage plates and to "cupping" of the metaphyses (Figs. 4-4 and 4-5).

Pathologic examination of a rachitic long bone, sectioned through the epiphysis and shaft (Fig. 4-3, *A*), or of a rib through the costochondral junction (Fig. 4-3, *B*), shows widening of the preparatory zone of cartilage (which may be irregularly invaded by perichondral and marrow vessels), lack of calcification of this cartilage (except perhaps in occasional small foci), and an irregular piling up of osteoid at the growth plate for lack of calcification and conversion to bone. The cortical and spongy tra-

65

beculae in the adjacent metaphysis may also be covered by osteoid. In severe rickets, the marrow may become somewhat fibrous.

Late rickets (rickets tarda). There are undoubtedly instances (Schmorl[23] and M. B. Schmidt) of rickets occurring late in childhood (from about 6 to 15 years of age) and attributable to dietary insufficiency. This is unusual, however, except under war starvation conditions. Such cases respond readily to treatment (Holt and Howland). The deformities are seldom extreme and the skeletal changes are most marked in the lower extremities.

Vitamin D—resistant rickets (hypophosphatemic—vitamin D refractory rickets; Debré-de Toni-Fanconi syndrome). There are occasional instances of more or less severe clinical rickets (Figs. 4-4 and 4-5) that require very large if not massive doses

of vitamin D for effective control. Dwarfing has been noted in such cases (de Toni). There also seems to be a history of familial incidence for this condition.

The prevailing view in regard to such cases is that the skeletal and other changes that develop are attributable to a defect in renal tubular reabsorption, whereby the kidneys leak phosphate, glucose, various amino acids, and possibly other metabolites.[29,30] Vitamin D—resistant rickets will be considered at greater length in Chapter 7.

Renal rickets (renal osteodystrophy). "Renal rickets" is an old, somewhat confusing designation for the rachitic skeletal changes (in a growing child) that develop as a result of secondary hyperparathyroidism complicating chronic renal insufficiency

Fig. 4-4. Roentgenograms showing the changes of vitamin D—resistant rickets.

Fig. 4-5. Another case of vitamin D—resistant rickets. Note the irregular widening of the growth zones and metaphyseal "cupping" at the distal radius and ulna.

of long standing (Fig. 4-6). This condition will also be discussed in Chapter 7.

Hypophosphatasia. Mention should be made of still another unusual condition, hypophosphatasia. In this disease skeletal changes resembling those of severe classical infantile rickets, or of osteomalacia in older patients, occur[35-37] for an entirely different reason. Failure to form bone by mineralization of osteoid at sites of endochondral ossification, and also to form adequate bone preformed in membrane in the calvarium, results not from lack of available bone-forming minerals but rather from failure of their utilization because of an inbred gene defect blocking the formation of the enzyme, phosphatase. Not only is there pronounced lowering of serum alkaline phosphatase activity, but there is also marked reduction of phosphatases in all tissues where they are ordinarily abundant. A survey of the literature on this disorder may be found in an article by Fraser.[35]

Osteomalacia. Osteomalacia, which must be distinguished from osteoporosis (Chapter 8), is the counterpart of rickets in adults or in any patients beyond the growth period. Like rickets, osteomalacia is characterized by a tendency to demineralization of the skeleton and by lack of adequate calcification of osteoid and its conversion thereby to bone.[38-40] Osteomalacia results from deficient absorption of calcium and/or phosphorus from the gut, or from their excessive excretion either in the stool or urine. While dietary deficiency may be the primary factor, this is comparatively rare under present conditions, at least in the United States. By far the most common causes are intestinal malabsorption, for whatever reason, and certain renal disorders.

To be sure, severe osteomalacia of the type found in women in India and China[41] after repeated child-bearing and lactation, on rations often deficient in vitamin D and bone-forming minerals, can lead to extreme skeletal demineralization and fantastic deformities of the pelvis, spine, and lower limb bones. After all, if far more calcium is used than is available, the deficit can come only from the skeleton. While osteomalacic bones have little tendency to break, if they get soft enough they can, under stress, bend like a pretzel. In the United States and in western Europe, one observes this only under extraordinary circumstances, such as war hunger or slow starvation, or in a few eccentric individuals on off-beat, vitamin-deficient diets. A notable example of hunger "osteopathy" or osteomalacia on a large scale was documented in Vienna during the lean years following World War I.[42] I have seen some of this abundant material at first hand from the pathologic collection of Professor

Fig. 4-6. Roentgenogram of the lower femora and tibiae of a child with secondary hyperparathyroidism associated with long-standing renal insufficiency—so-called renal rickets.

Fig. 4-7. **A,** Roentgenogram of an adult with osteomalacia. Note the uniform thinning of the cortices and the transverse pseudofractures in the upper tibiae and fibulae. **B,** The upper femur of the same patient as in **A.**

Fig. 4-8. Roentgenogram of a patient with osteomalacia who also presented multiple, spontaneous, symmetrical pseudofractures.

Erdheim, and the preparations show exquisite osteomalacia.

Perhaps the most common cause of early or less severe forms of osteomalacia found in adults today (and this disease is by no means unusual) is intestinal malabsorption.[43] This may be associated with bypassing gastrointestinal operations, pancreatitis,[44] the steatorrhea of nontropical sprue,[45,46] or such intestinal disorders as regional enteritis or Whipple's disease. It would appear that the poor absorption of calcium and phosphorus in these circumstances is as important for the development of osteomalacia as the malabsorption of fat-soluble vitamin D, if not more so.

The other common cause of osteomalacia is renal disorder characterized by excessive urinary excretion of phosphate.[47] As previously noted, the congenital disorder of tubular transport of phosphate, glucose, and amino acids, described by Debré and de Toni[48] and later by Fanconi, can lead to osteomalacia as well as rickets. It must be kept in mind, however, that hyperphosphaturia per se can also reflect parathyroid hyperplasia developing in response to hypocalcemia.

Whatever the cause of osteomalacia, appreciable thinning and rarefaction of bone cortices eventually ensue. Associated with this are generalized bone tenderness, bowing, compression of vertebral bodies, and, rather characteristically, Looser zones[49] and painful symmetrical transverse fissure pseudofractures (so-called Milkman's syndrome).[50] The latter may be seen in the shafts of long limb bones (Fig. 4-7) and in such sites as the medial border of the scapula and the inferior ramus of the pubis.[51]

As for significant serum chemical changes, the calcium or the phosphorus level is on the low side; in advanced cases, both may be markedly reduced. The serum alkaline phosphatase activity is consistently elevated. Tubular reabsorption of phosphate is high early in the course of the disease, and low later on, when hypocalcemia has led to secondary hyperparathyroidism.

Biopsy of an affected bone or of the iliac crest in osteomalacia may present a complex picture in advanced cases, with their overlay of stress reaction and secondary hyperparathyroidism. The basic diagnostic feature, however, apart from thinning of cortical bone, is the finding of osteoid borders on the bone trabeculae. These are seen to best advantage after very slow decalcification (several weeks) in Müller's fluid. After the customary rapid decalcification with acid or a chelating agent, it may be difficult to distinguish the osteoid seams clearly from the underlying bone. We have found it helpful to use acridine orange stain and ultraviolet light microscopy.

Osteomalacia can be cured, with restoration of skeletal function, by the administration of large doses of vitamin D, but therapy must be tailored to fit the individual patient. At times, as much as 1,000,000 units per day may be required. Care should be taken to prevent overdose with its hazards of hypercalcemia and nephrocalcinosis. It is self-evident also that an adequate source of calcium must be provided in the diet and that the deleterious effects of the underlying intestinal or renal disorder must be ameliorated if at all possible. With good clinical management and avoidance of vitamin D overdosage, pseudofractures become calcified and the bones become denser, although the bowing deformities persist and may require osteotomy

for correction.[52] It is possible that the availability of 25-hydroxycholecalciferol (25-HCC), a more potent, active form of vitamin D, will make clinical management easier.

Vitamin D excess or poisoning (*hypervitaminosis D*)

As in the case of vitamin A, too much of a good thing—in this case vitamin D—can be harmful, if not dangerous. Hypervitaminosis D results from the administration of excessive or massive doses of vitamin D in one form or another, ostensibly with therapeutic intent. There was a spate of such cases some years ago[31-33] before the toxicity of excessive vitamin D was recognized. The substance was used (or commercially exploited) in the treatment of rheumatoid arthritis, as well as other conditions. In these circumstances, there is a significant increase in the serum calcium level, up to 12 or 16 mg. or more, presumably the result of increased absorption of calcium from the gut.

The two major manifestations of vitamin D poisoning are: (1) the usual untoward effects of marked hypercalcemia, and (2) widespread calcific deposits, sometimes massive, in many sites throughout the body, both skeletal (joints) and visceral. Those in the kidneys (nephrocalcinosis) may be potentially serious. If the condition persists long enough, demineralization of the skeleton ensues, although the mechanism for this is not altogether clear. The obvious therapeutic measures are cessation of vitamin D administration, a low calcium diet, abundant fluid intake to flush out the kidneys, and the administration of corticoids to reduce hypercalcemia.[34]

References

1. Blackfan, K. D., and Wolbach, S. B.: Vitamin A deficiency in infants: clinical and pathological study, J. Pediat. 3:679, 1933.
2. Bass, M. H., and Caplan, J.: Vitamin A deficiency in infancy, J. Pediat. 67:690, 1955.
3. Cornfeld, D., and Cooke, R. E.: Vitamin A

deficiency: case report, unusual manifestations in 5½ month old baby, Pediatrics **10**:33, 1952.

4. Wolbach, J. B.: Vitamin A deficiency and excess in relation to skeletal growth, J. Bone Joint Surg. **29**:171, 1947.

5. Wolf, I. J.: Vitamin A deficiency in an infant, J.A.M.A. **166**:1859, 1958.

6. Maxwell, J. P.: Vitamin deficiency in antenatal period: its effect on mother and infant, J. Obstet. Gynaec. Brit. Comm. **39**:764, 1932.

7. Warkany, J., and Nelson, R. C.: The appearance of skeletal abnormalities in the offspring of rats reared on a deficient diet, Science **92**:383, 1940.

8. Wilson, J. G., and Barch, S.: Fetal death and maldevelopment resulting from maternal vitamin A deficiency in the rat, Proc. Soc. Exp. Biol. Med. **72**:687, 1949.

9. Josephs, H. W.: Hypervitaminosis A and carotinemia, Amer. J. Dis. Child. **67**:33, 1944.

10. Caffey, J.: Chronic poisoning due to excess of vitamin A: description of clinical and roentgen manifestations in seven infants and young children, Pediatrics **5**:672, 1950.

11. Fried, C. T., and Grand, M. J.: Hypervitaminosis A, Amer. J. Dis. Child. **79**:475, 1950.

12. Cohlan, S. Q.: Excessive intake of vitamin A as a cause of congenital anomalies in the rat, Science **117**:535, 1953.

13. Moore, T., and Wang, Y. L.: Hypervitaminosis A, Biochem. J. **399**:222, 1945.

14. Rodahl, K.: Hypervitaminosis A, Norske Polarinstitut, Skrifter Nr. **95**:73, 1950.

15. Weissmann, G., Bell, E., and Thomas, L.: Prevention by hydrocortisone of changes in connective tissue induced by an excess of vitamin A, Amer. J. Path. **42**:571, 1963.

16. Hess, A. F.: Scurvy, past and present, Philadelphia, 1920, J. B. Lippincott Co.

17. Barlow, T.: On cases described as acute rickets, Med. Clin. Trans. **66**:159, 1883.

18. Holt, H., and Frolich, T.: Ueber experimentallen Skorbut, Z. Hyg. Infektionskr. **72**:1, 1912.

19. Lauman, T. H., and Ingalls, T. H.: Vitamin C deficiency and wound healing, Ann. Surg. **105**:616, 1937.

20. McCallum, W. G.: A text-book of pathology, ed. 3, Philadelphia, 1924, W. B. Saunders Co., pp. 927-929.

21. Follis, R. H., Jr.: Histochemical studies on cartilage and bone; ascorbic acid deficiency, Bull. Johns Hopk. Hosp. **89**:9, 1951.

22. Wolbach, S. B., and Howe, P. R.: Intercellular substance in experimental scorbutus, Arch Path. Lab. Med. **1**:1, 1926.

23. Schmorl, G.: Ergebn. Inn. Med. Kinderheilk. **4**:403, 1909.

24. Hess, A. F.: Rickets including osteomalacia and tetany, Philadelphia, 1929, Lea & Febiger.

25. Mellanby, E.: An experimental investigation on rickets, Lancet **1**:407, 1919.

26. Pappenheimer, A. M.: Anatomical changes accompanying healing experimental rat rickets under influence of cod liver oil or its active derivatives, J. Exp. Med. **36**:335, 1922.

27. Park, E. A.: Etiology of rickets, Physiol. Rev. **3**:106, 1923.

28. Richards, I. D. G., Sweet, E. M., and Arneil, G. C.: Infantile rickets persists in Glasgow, Lancet **1**:7546, 1968.

29. Tapia, J., Stearns, G., and Ponseti, I. V.: Vitamin D resistant rickets; a long-term clinical study of 11 patients, J. Bone Joint Surg. **46-A**:935, 1964.

30. Winters, R. W., Graham, J. B., Williams, T. F., McFalls, V. W., and Burnett, C. H.: A genetic study of familial hypophosphatemia and vitamin D resistant rickets with a review of the literature, Medicine **37**:97, 1958.

31. Adams, F. D.: Reversible uremia with hypercalcemia due to vitamin D intoxication, New Eng. J. Med. **244**:590, 1951.

32. Chaplin, H., Clark, L. D., and Ropes, M. W.: Vitamin D intoxication, Amer. J. Med. Sci. **221**:369, 1951.

33. Christensen, W. R., Liebman, C., and Sosman, M. C.: Skeletal and periarticular manifestations of hypervitaminosis D, Amer. J. Roentgen. **65**:27, 1951.

34. Verner, J., and others: Vitamin D intoxication and report of 2 cases treated with cortisone, Ann. Intern. Med. **48**:765, 1958.

35. Fraser, R.: Amer. J. Med. **22**:730, 1957.

36. Bethune, J. E., and Dent, C. E.: Hypophosphatasia in the adult, Amer. J. Med. **28**:615, 1960.

37. Kellsey, D. C.: Hypophosphatasia and congenital bowing of the long bones, J.A.M.A. **179**:187, 1962.

38. Albright, F., Burnett, C. H., Parson, W., Reifenstein, E. C., and Roos, A.: Osteomalacia and late rickets, Medicine **25**:399, 1946.

39. Engle, R. L., and Wallis, L. A.: Amer. J. Med. **22**:5-13, 1957.

40. McCrudden, F. M.: Studies in bone metabolism and osteomalacia, Arch. Intern. Med. **5**:596, 1910.

41. Maxwell, J. P.: Osteomalacia in China, China Med. J. **38**:349, 1924.

42. Dalyell, E. S., and Chick, H.: Hunger-osteomalacia in Vienna, 1920, Lancet **2**:842, 1921.

43. Picchi, J., Crane, J., Gordan, G. S., Sakai, H. Q., and Steinbach, H.: Parathyroid function in malabsorption osteomalacia, Clin. Res. Proc. **5**:67, 1957.

44. Plough, I. C., and Kyle, L. H.: Pancreatic insufficiency and hyperparathyroidism, Ann. Intern. Med. **47**:590, 1957.

45. Dent, C. E.: Hyperparathyroidism and steatorrhea, Brit. Med. J. **2**:1546, 1956.

46. Fraser, R., and Nordin, B. E. C.: Hyperparathyroidism and steatorrhea, Brit. Med. J. **2**:1363, 1956.

47. Dent, C. E.: Rickets and ostetomalacia from renal tubule defects, J. Bone Joint Surg. **34-B**:266, 1952.

48. De Toni, G.: Renal rickets with phospho- gluco-amino renal diabetes (de Toni-Debre-Fanconi syndrome), Ann. Paediat. **187**:42, 1956.

49. Looser, E.: Über pathologicsche form von Infraktionen und Callusbildungen bei Rachitis und Osteomalacie und anderen Knochenerkrankungen, Zbl. Chir. **47**:1470, 1920.

50. Milkman, L. A.: Multiple spontaneous idiopathic symmetrical fractures, Amer. J. Roentgen. **32**:622, 1934.

51. Steinbach, H. L., Kolb, F. O., and Gilfillan, R.: A mechanism of the production of pseudo-fractures in osteomalacia (Milkman's syndrome), Radiology **62**:388, 1954.

52. Gordan, G. S.: Osteomalacia: diagnosis and treatment, Texas State J. Med. **59**:110, 1963.

Chapter 5

Skeletal changes in endocrine disorders

In this highly active subspecialty of internal medicine and pediatrics, there are available a number of commendable monographs and otherwise a vast literature to which many gifted clinical investigators have contributed. Each new annual *Year Book of Endocrinology* directs attention to hundreds of relevant new observations. For me to attempt anything more than a thumbnail sketch of the skeletal changes found in the well-recognized disorders of the various endocrine glands resulting from hypo- or hyperfunction would be impractical as well as presumptuous.

Pituitary gland

Pituitary basophilism (basophil cell adenoma of the anterior lobe) was at one time thought by Cushing (1932) to be responsible for the clinical entity or syndrome that bears his name, although it is now recognized that this explanation is valid in relatively few instances. Even in these, the untoward effects may well be mediated through stimulation of excessive adrenal cortical activity. As indicated in Chapter 8, one of the major features of *Cushing's syndrome* is pronounced osteoporosis, manifested clinically in backache, round shoulders, and multiple fractures, especially of the ribs.

Hyperfunction of the eosinophil cells of the anterior lobe, resulting from either diffuse hyperplasia or adenoma, has a very striking effect on skeletal growth. If the condition has its onset before puberty, *pituitary gigantism* results (Fig. 5-1). Persons with this condition are the 7- to 8-foot circus giants, whose exaggerated skeletal growth reflects inordinate stimulation of endochondral ossification or its reactivation. Other related manifestations are hypertrophy of the subcutaneous tissues and a tendency to periosteal new bone deposition, readily apparent on the jaw bones, for example.

If, on the other hand, the condition develops after the growth period, the condition of *acromegaly* (Fig. 5-2) is the result. This condition features the familiar thickset appearance, coarse face, narrow barrel chest with dorsal kyphosis (from reactivated growth at costochondral junctions), large joints, massive hands and feet with thickened digits, and conspicuous prognathism (lantern jaw).[1-7] The skull changes associated with prominent enlargement of the head are particularly noteworthy: balloon-like expansion of the sella turcica, great increase in the angle of the mandible with resulting malocclusion and separation of teeth, thickening of the calvarium, over-development of the frontal sinuses and mastoids, and pronounced enlargement of the external occipital protuberance. Other parts of the skeleton, including the vertebral column, show comparable enlargement, particularly at sites of muscle attachment, while the spade-like hand bones show tufting of the terminal phalanges. In long-standing acromegaly, joint changes not unlike those of hypertrophic osteoarthritis eventually ensue, although their pathogenesis is somewhat different.

Fig. 5-1. Pituitary gigantism. Note feeble, eunuchoid appearance and hypotrichosis of patient, whose height was over 8 feet. (From Lisser, H., and Escamilla, R. F.: Atlas of clinical endocrinology, ed. 2, St. Louis, 1961, The C. V. Mosby Co.)

| A | B | C |

Fig. 5-2. A, Acromegalic patient showing protruding sternum, kyphosis, heavy coarse features, and prognathus. B and C, Comparison of acromegalic hand and foot with those of a normal adult male (on the right of each figure). (From Lisser, H., and Escamilla, R. F.: Atlas of clinical endocrinology, ed. 2, St. Louis, 1962, The C. V. Mosby Co.)

Hypopituitarism, caused most often by tumors of the craniopharyngeal duct or Rathke's pouch, results during childhood in the *Lorain type of dwarfism* (nanosomia pituitaria in the old terminology of Erdheim[8]), which is characterized by somatic underdevelopment, stunting of growth, and sexual immaturity (Fig. 5-3). The body habitus is featured by slender fragile build, thin skin, and very fine hair. As in hypothyroidism, there is significant delay in the appearance and ossification of epiph-

Fig. 5-3. Hypophyseal infantilism. Girl on the left, age 15, is sexually infantile. Her normal sister, on the right, is 2 years younger and well matured. Patient's height was only 3 feet, 9 inches. Bone age was estimated as 10 years. This patient presents a striking example of pituitary dwarfism plus sexual infantilism. (From Lisser, H., and Escamilla, R. F.: Atlas of clinical endocrinology, ed. 2, St. Louis, 1962, The C. V. Mosby Co.)

yses. Administration of pituitary growth hormone extracted from human glands obtained fresh at autopsy has proved to be of therapeutic value in the hands of Li and his associates[9] at the University of California. Hopefully, we shall one day have a potent synthetic product available for general use.

In male adolescents or preadolescents, the *Fröhlich* type of plumpness and girdle-like adiposity *(dystrophia adiposogenitalis)* is associated with somatic and skeletal underdevelopment. There is also characteristic loss of sexual libido and potency.

Complete destruction of the anterior lobe of the pituitary, whatever its cause, is incompatible with life and leads to an eventually fatal cachectic state (Simmond's disease).

Adrenal glands

With reference to skeletal changes particularly, mention should be made here of *hypercorticism* as seen in Cushing's syndrome,[10-12] which results in marked thinning of the bones, among other familiar effects. The catabolic effect on bone of excessive adrenal corticoids, whether these are produced by tumorous or hyperplastic suprarenal glands or are administered therapeutically, will be discussed in Chapter 8.

Benign or malignant cortical tumors may have other relevant effects, stemming from the fact that the adrenal cortex normally elaborates a significant quantity of androgenic hormones. In the female, these hormones generally have a masculinizing effect; in the male, exaggerated male characteristics become manifest. In the male child, sexual precocity and inordinate muscular development in these circumstances make for a little Hercules. The skeleton shows acceleration of growth at first, but the end result paradoxically is premature fusion of epiphyses and small stature. In the adolescent or adult male, a condition of virility and striking hirsutism may result.

Fig. 5-4. Roentgenograms showing delayed skeletal development in a young patient with cretinism.

Thyroid gland

Hyperthyroidism (Graves' disease, Basedow's disease, exophthalmic goiter) may sometimes induce skeletal demineralization leading to clinical osteoporosis, involving the calvarium, ribs, and spine. Concomitantly, there is increased urinary excretion of calcium and phosphorus. If prolonged and untreated, the demineralization of bone can be as pronounced as that in Cushing's syndrome. If the onset of the condition is before the end of adolescence, there may be accelerated skeletal growth.

Protracted, untreated *hypothyroidism* leads to myxedema in the adult and to *cretinism* in young children. One of the manifestations of cretinism is dwarfism, which may result from congenital aplasia of the thyroid, from subtotal inflammatory or infectious destruction of the gland, or from endemic iodine deficiency (in mountainous regions). Occasionally it can result from one of a series of inherited enzymatic disorders of thyroid hormone synthesis. What-

ever the cause, there is delayed appearance and retarded growth of centers of ossification (Fig. 5-4), retarded growth at epiphyseal cartilage plates, and persistence of growth plates and sutures beyond their usual age of disappearance and even into adult life. Eventually, deformities of the articular ends of long bones may ensue.

Mention should also be made here of *thyrocalcitonin,* discovered by Copp in 1963. Thyrocalcitonin is a hormone secreted by the thyroid gland (independently of the parathyroids) that plays a role in calcium homeostasis. It has been stated that it is responsible for incorporation of calcium into bone and that it can actively lower the serum calcium and block bone resorption (essentially the reverse of the parathyroid effect on bone). The hormone has been successfully synthesized by several pharmaceutical teams, and one can therefore look forward to early exploration of its clinical effects and therapeutic application.

Gonads

Primary hypogonadism, whether it results from castration, trauma, or infection, has no effect on the skeleton when it develops after the growth period, except insofar as it may favor osteoporosis (in women). In female children with *ovarian agenesis,* stunted growth or *dwarfism,* which is often associated with other congenital developmental anomalies such as webbed neck or coarctation of the aorta, is found. Hypogonadism in the male child results in *eunuchism* or eunuchoid habitus, depending upon its degree. The skeleton is relatively tall, the limb bones are long and slender with thin cortices, and the epiphyseal cartilage plates persist beyond the normal age and remain active.

Pineal gland

Teratomas of the pineal gland and, less often, pinealomas encroaching on the third ventricle and invading the hypothalamus may be responsible in young male children for the *macrogenitosomia praecox* syndrome. As its name implies, this syndrome is featured by excessive body growth and genital development and other manifestations of precocious puberty. The skeleton shows advanced centers of ossification, so that the long bones, for example, are large and heavy in relation to the age of the subject.

Pancreas

Hypofunction of islet tissue resulting in clinical *diabetes mellitus* may be responsible for altered skeletal development in children. Specifically, with recent onset of the disease, the centers of ossification may be advanced so that initially the body height is above average for the age of the patient. However, with a long history, the centers of ossification may eventually be retarded; the bones are then thin and narrow and even osteoporotic.

In adults, one may see accelerated arteriosclerosis with narrowing and occlusion of peripheral arteries, as well as a tendency to gangrene and infection, particularly in the lower limbs. Also noteworthy is the yellow-brown discoloration of the bones, especially of the calvarium, to which Schmorl directed attention many years ago.

Thymus

As Rowntree and his associates demonstrated, injection of potent thymic extract into young animals (rats) can bring about accelerated prepubertal growth and development, hastened onset of adolescence in the offspring, and increased fertility of parent animals. This is, of course, of more theoretic than practical importance.

Parathyroid glands

Primary hyperparathyroidism has received a tremendous amount of attention in recent years. Diagnosis of this condition is now made more often and much earlier, before irreversible renal damage from stone formation or nephrocalcinosis has developed. To make an early diagnosis, one must be alert and resourceful and have available a consistently accurate biochemical laboratory.

Clinical leads to diagnosis may be urolithiasis or nephrocalcinosis, symptoms of acute hypercalcemia (nausea, vomiting, constipation, weight loss, anorexia, abdominal pain, refractory peptic ulcer, muscular weakness, and psychosis), or evidence of skeletal resorptive changes (from knowledgeable roentgenographic examination, tracer studies of bone mineral turnover, and bone biopsy). In the presence of hypercalcemia, serum protein electrophoretic separation (showing elevation of $alpha_2$ and beta globulins) will help to rule out other conditions, such as myeloma or sarcoidosis, which may also be characterized by hypercalcemia.

It is noteworthy also that the hypercalcemia of hyperparathyroidism does not respond to large doses of cortisone, as does frequently the hypercalcemia of malig-

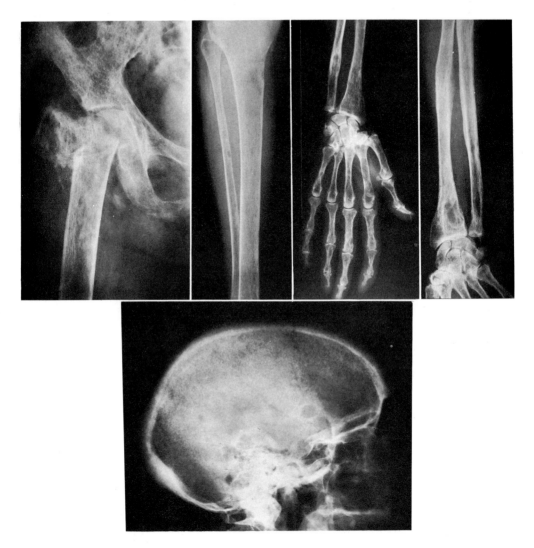

Fig. 5-5. Roentgenograms illustrating delayed recognition of hyperparathyroidism in a 60-year-old woman whose initial manifestation was fracture of the hip. This went on to nonunion after nailing, and two reconstructive procedures in the course of the next 10 months were also unsuccessful. Pain in the wrist area directed attention to the presence of circumscribed lucent defects in the distal radius and other sites, and skeletal survey showed appreciable cortical thining of the limb bones and granular porosity of the calvarium. Biopsy of the lesion in the radius pointed to hyperparathyroidism, and the serum calcium level was 16 mg. On surgical exploration (performed 15 months after fracture of the hip) a chief cell parathyroid adenoma was found, the cytology of which is illustrated in Fig. 5-10.

Fig. 5-6. Roentgenogram of another patient with hyperparathyroidism, showing multiple lytic defects in both innominate bones ("brown tumors"), one of which protruded from the ilium.

Fig. 5-7. A, From another case of proved hyperparathyroidism, in which a striking feature was the finding of a large "brown tumor" in the proximal radius. **B,** Reossification of the lesion in **A** 4 years after removal of the parathyroid tumor; the expansion and deformity of the bone persisted.

A   **B**

Fig. 5-8. Another instance of delayed recognition of hyperparathyroidism in a 57-year-old woman whose presenting skeletal lesion in an ulna (with pain and swelling) was taken to be a giant cell tumor and resected as such. Subsequently, lucent defects were found in other bones and the serum calcium level was noted to be 14.5 mg. On exploration of the neck, a parathyroid adenoma was found. **A,** Roentgenogram of the resected portion of the ulnar bone showing expansion, marked thinning of the cortex, and cyst-like rarefaction of the bone throughout. **B,** Photograph of half of the specimen illustrating cortical thinning, reddish discoloration, and cystic transformation of its interior.

nancy, hyperthyroidism, sarcoidosis, vitamin D intoxication, Addison's disease, and so forth. In addition to persistent hypercalcemia, renal phosphate leak must also be demonstrated for the correct preoperative diagnosis of hyperparathyroidism. For this, measurement of the tubular reabsorption of phosphorus (TRP) has been proved to be reliable by Gordan, Eisenberg, and their associates.[13-15]

Roentgenographic skeletal examination is also a valuable aid in diagnosis. In the large series surveyed by Steinbach,[15] some 22% of cases of subsequently proved hyperparathyroidism showed significant subperiosteal resorption of the cortex, best seen on the radial surface of the index and middle fingers. Some of these patients also showed granular mottling of bone elsewhere, notably in the calvarium; others showed localized rarefaction defects at the site of "brown tumors." Diffuse demineralization is not necessarily to be expected, although it may be a prominent feature; nor is resorption of the lamina dura of the teeth as dependable a criterion as was once thought (Figs. 5-5 to 5-8).

Bone involvement can be demonstrated in many additional patients with hyperparathyroidism by tracer studies (using nonradioactive strontium, for example) and by bone biopsy. In all these instances one may expect to find elevated serum alkaline phosphatase activity. However, there are undoubtedly cases of proved hyperparathyroidism in which biopsy (of the iliac crest) fails to show evidence of resorption. Perhaps this reflects early sophisticated clinical diagnosis and effective surgery, as contrasted with the bygone era in which the commonly observed end stage of long-standing osseous involvement was the devastating picture of "generalized osteitis fibrosa cystica," as described by von Recklinghausen in 1891.

When bone biopsy does show mild porosity and focal resorption tracts on spongy trabeculae or around enlarged vessel canals in the cortex, these are not pathognomonic, inasmuch as they may also be found in other conditions such as chronic renal insufficiency with uremia, breast cancer, and osteomalacia. All that the pathologist can and should say is that the changes observed are consistent with hyperparathyroidism, which is essentially a clinical diagnosis, at least prior to surgery.

Occasionally the pathologist has the opportunity to examine material from a *brown tumor,* operated, as likely as not, because it was thought radiographically and clinically to be a giant cell tumor, an aneurysmal bone cyst, or perhaps a benign tumor of undetermined nature, before the presence of hypercalcemia was ascertained. The concept of the so-called brown tumor is also a relic of an old era in pathology— it is neither brown (but red, before fixation) nor a tumor. It represents essentially a localized area of exaggerated skeletal resorption, appearing radiographically as a circumscribed lucent defect of varying size and location (the jaw bones, calvarium, and hand bones may be affected, as well as long bones). Its distinction pathologically from giant cell tumor of bone is a subtle one at times, but it can be made with reasonable assurance by an experienced observer. Suffice it to state here that the lesion of hyperparathyroidism has a more fibrous stroma and shows some new bone formation as a rule, as an expression of attempted reconstruction. Further, its giant cells are of the nature of macrophages (rather than syncytial tumor cells), lodged for the most part within or close to vascular channels and appearing in response to blood extravasation (Figs. 5-8, *B,* and 5-9).

As for the changes in the parathyroids themselves, these have been thoroughly explored by Castleman and others on the basis of extensive material. In the great majority of instances of primary hyperparathyroidism, a single parathyroid adenoma is found (Fig. 5-10); only occasionally is more than one encountered. In a mi-

Fig. 5-9. **A,** Photomicrograph of a "brown tumor" in hyperparathyroidism. Note resorption and fibrous replacement of bone, slight new bone formation, and concentration of giant cell macrophages at a site of blood extravasation. **B,** A field from a "brown tumor" showing the osteoclast-like macrophages lodged within thin-walled vascular channels. This picture is quite different from that of neoplastic giant cell tumor of bone.

nority of cases (about 10% or less), there may be hypertrophy and hyperplasia of all four parathyroid glands. Only rarely is hyperparathyroidism caused by a carcinoma (although certain tumors elsewhere may cause hypercalcemia).

On the other hand, in parathyroid hyperplasia secondary to renal disease or osteomalacia, for example, all the glands are regularly enlarged. Some other less common causes of parathyroid enlargement are Paget's disease, metastatic carcinoma, myeloma, and Cushing's syndrome. The subject of secondary hyperparathyroidism, at least in relation to its most frequent causes, has been considered elsewhere (see sections on renal disease, rickets, and osteomalacia). For the sake of brevity, the observations made will not be reiterated here.

Hypoparathyroidism. Hypoparathyroidism results most often after inadvertent removal of several parathyroid glands in the course of thyroidectomy; it is less often idiopathic or spontaneous, reflecting aplasia or atrophy of the glands. It may also develop temporarily after parathyroidectomy (for adenoma); this must be anticipated. As one might expect from the dual effect of the parthyroid hormone, the serum calcium level is low (at tetany level), while the serum phosphorus level is elevated and the tubular reabsorption of phosphorus is correspondingly high.

The major clinical manifestations relate to tetany (epilepsy or brain tumor may be simulated), cataract formation, calcification of basal ganglia, and mental deterioration (with inadequate treatment). In hypoparathyroidism of long standing, stunting of stature and a variety of other skeletal changes have been described.

Effective therapy is directed toward rais-

Fig. 5-10. Photomicrograph showing chief cell hyperplasia in the parathyroid adenoma removed in the case illustrated in Fig. 5-5.

ing the blood calcium level by ingestion of calcium salts and/ or administration of vitamin D, and toward lowering the phosphate level by avoidance of phosphate-rich foods, by ingestion of aluminum hydroxide to adsorb phosphate in the gut, and by administration of vitamin D or dihydrotachysterol. The administration of parathyroid extract is not favored, since this relatively crude protein product may lead to refractoriness.

In *pseudo-hypoparathyroidism*, the symptoms are caused not by deficiency in the glands themselves but rather by failure of the renal tubule to respond to the phosphuretic action of parathyroid hormone. In such subjects, short stature, brachydactyly, and foci of subcutaneous calcification have been described.

Pseudo-pseudo-hypoparathyroidism denotes a variant of pseudo-hypoparathyroidism in which characteristic bone changes are absent.[16]

Finally, to confound the inexpert reader even more, there have been a number of recent case reports[16-18] on coexistence of both diminished and increased parathyroid function. This condition has been paradoxically designated *hypo-hyperparathyroidism*.

References

1. Atkinson, F. R. B.: Acromegaly, London, 1932, John Bale Sons & Danielsson.
2. Bailey, P.: Intracranial tumors, Springfield, Illinois, 1933, Charles C Thomas, Publisher.
3. Cushing, H.: Pituitary body and its disorders, Philadelphia, 1912, J. B. Lippincott Co.
4. Erdheim, J.: Über Wirbelsaülenveränderungen bei Akromegalie, Virch. Arch. Path. Anat. 281:197, 1931.
5. Marie, P.: Sur deux cas d'acromégalie, Rev. Méd. 6:297, 1886.
6. Marie, P., and Marinesco, G.: Sur l'anatomie pathologique de l'acromégalie, Arch. Méd. Exp. Anat. Path. 3:539, 1891.
7. Virchow, R.: Ein Fall und ein skelet von Akromegalie, Klin. Wschr. 26:81, 1889.
8. Erdheim, J.: Nanosomia pituitaria, Beitr. Path. Anat. 62:302, 1916.
9. Li, C. H., and Papkoff, H.: Preparation and properties for growth hormone from human and monkey pituitary glands, Science 124: 1293, 1956.
10. Knowlton, A. J.: Cushing's syndrome, Bull. N.Y. Acad. Med. 29:441, 1953.
11. Poutasse, E. F., and Higgins, C. C.: Surgery of the adrenal gland for Cushing's syndrome, J. Urol. 70:129, 1953.
12. Strickland, B.: Cushing's syndrome, Proc. Roy. Soc. Med. 47:341, 1954.
13. Gordan, G. S.: Hyperparathyroidism, Texas State J. Med. 57:578, 1961.
14. Gordan, G. S., Eisenberg, E., Loken, H. F., Gardner, B., and Hayashida, T.: Clinical endocrinology of parathyroid hormone excess, Recent Progr. Hormone Res. 18:297, 1962.
15. Steinbach, H. L., Gordan, G. S., Eisenberg, E., Crane, J. T., Silverman, S., and Goldman, L.: Primary hyperparathyroidism: a correlation of roentgen, clinical and pathological features, Amer. J. Roentgen. 86:329, 1961.
16. Editorial: Pity the twisting tongue, J.A.M.A. 205:92, 1968.
17. Costello, J. M., and Dent, C. E.: Hypo-hyperparathyroidism, Arch. Dis. Child. 38:397, 1963.
18. Watson, L.: Hypo-hyperparathyroidism, Proc. Roy. Soc. Med. 61:287, 1968.

General references

Albright, F., Burnett, C. H., Smith, P. H., and Parson, W.: Pseudo-hypoparathyroidism—example of "Seabright-bantam syndrome"; report of 3 cases, Endocrinology 30:922, 1942.

Albright, F., Smith, P. H., and Fraser, R.: A syndrome characterized by primary ovarian insufficiency and decreased stature, Amer. J. Med. Sci. 204:625, 1942.

Bortz, W., and others: Differentiation between thyroid and and parathyroid causes of hypercalcemia, Ann. Intern. Med. 54:610, 1961.

Dent, C.: Some problems of hyperparathyroidism, Brit. Med. J. 2:1419, 1962.

Hellstrom, J., and others: Primary hyperparathyroidism, Acta Chir. Scand. 294 (Supp.):1-113, 1962.

Jailer, J. W.: Virilism, Bull. N. Y. Acad. Med. 29:377, 1953.

Kolb, F. O., and Steinbach, H.: Pseudohyperparathyroidism with secondary hyperparathyroidism and osteitis fibrosa, J. Clin. Endocr. 22:59, 1962.

Rasmussen, H.: Parathyroid hormone: nature and mechanism of action, Amer. J. Med. 30:112, 1961.

Rasmussen, H., and Reifenstein, E. C., Jr.: The parathyroid glands. In Williams, R. H., editor:

Textbook of endocrinology, ed. 3, Philadelphia, 1962, W. B. Saunders Co., pp. 731-879.

Robinson, P. K., Carmichael, E. A., and Cumings, J. N.: Idiopathic hypoparathyroidism; study of 3 cases, Quart. J. Med. 23:383, 1954.

Wilkins, L.: The diagnosis and treatment of endocrine disorders in childhood and adolescence, Springfield, Illinois, 1965, Charles C Thomas, Publisher.

Wilkins, L.: Disturbances in growth, Bull. N. Y. Acad. Med. 29:280, 1953.

Wilkins, L. and Fleischmann, W.: The diagnosis of hypothyroidism in childhood, J.A.M.A. 116:2459, 1941.

Chapter 6

Skeletal changes in metabolic disorders

This chapter will deal mainly with an assortment of conditions that have in common the fact that they result from inborn errors of metabolism. These conditions are bracketed here for convenient orientation. The main groupings, considered mainly for their skeletal effects, are: the primary disorders of lipid metabolism (especially Gaucher's disease and xanthoma tuberosum multiplex), disorders of purine metabolism (gout, in particular), abnormal amino acid metabolism (especially hereditary ochronosis, which produces significant bone and joint disease), abnormal mucopolysaccharide metabolism (gargoylism is the major condition in point), and some disorders of pigment metabolism (porphyria, mainly). Also considered briefly will be miscellaneous conditions such as amyloidosis, the effect of cachetic states on the bone marrow, and the influence of trace elements on the skeleton.

The skeletal changes in some other important metabolic disorders, most of which are not congenital, have been discussed in other chapters. For the sake of brevity, these observations will not be reiterated here. Specifically, these conditions are scurvy, rickets, and osteomalacia (discussed in Chapter 4); diabetes mellitus (Chapter 5); chronic renal insufficiency,

with or without secondary hyperparathyroidism (Chapters 4, 5, and 7); aminoaciduria and other manifestations of renal tubular transport disease (Chapter 7); and sprue, steatorrhea, and pancreatic insufficiency (Chapter 4).

Primary disorders of lipid metabolism

After being dormant for a long time, lipid metabolism has once again become the subject of active investigation. As additional observations accrue, the disorders in question become increasingly complex. Thus Niemann-Pick disease, once thought to be a lethal disease of young infants,[1] is now believed to occur in adults as well.[2-4] Collaterally, relatively new concepts of systemic infantile lipoidosis (generalized gangliosidosis[5,6]) and of mucopolysaccharidosis have developed. Gaucher's disease, once considered to be a protracted disease of adults,[7,8] is now recognized as occurring occasionally in a more acute form in infants and young children.[9,10] Amaurotic idiocy, once thought to be an entity of uniform character (Tay-Sachs disease), is now held to appear in no less than six recognized clinical types, according to Volk,[5,6] that affect older patients as well as infants.

As for familial hyperlipoproteinemia and the problems of fat transport by lipoproteins in general,[12] at least five different patterns of circulating lipids of varying clinical significance are now recognized, reflecting increases in the chylomicron, cholesterol, beta lipoprotein, and triglyceride fractions, respectively. While these observations are of great interest to geneticists, pediatricians, and biochemists, as well as internists concerned with the clinical management of arteriosclerosis, the brief account in this book must, of necessity, be limited to the meaningful skeletal alterations that may ensue.

Niemann-Pick disease. In Niemann-Pick disease, prominent aggregates of foam cells are found at autopsy[1] in the bone marrow, in the other reticulum-bearing organs, and in many other sites throughout the body (lungs, intestine, kidneys, and so on). As a rule, there are no structural changes in affected bones (as there may be in Gaucher's disease), perhaps because the condition does not last long enough for them to develop.

Gaucher's disease. Gaucher's disease is another congenital, and sometimes familial, disorder of lipid metabolism. It is characterized by excessive widespread deposition of a glucocerebroside long designated as kerasin,[13] notably in the spleen (which can become huge), in the liver (which may eventually undergo cirrhosis), in the bones (which undergo certain structural alterations, infarcts, and, occasionally, fractures), in the deeper lymph nodes, and, to a lesser extent, in other structures such as the skin and conjunctivae. Presumably, the condition results from a gene or enzyme defect, as do inbred disorders of metabolism generally. However, analytic lipid chemistry is so complex that it may be some time before the precise nature of the block in the relevant metabolic pathway is ascertained.[14]

Whatever its site of deposition, kerasin is taken up by aggregates of distinctive large, pale, foamy histiocytes with delicate fibrillar striations within their cytoplasm;

these are quite different from ordinary foam cells containing cholesterol esters. In fact, their appearance is pathognomonic of Gaucher's disease. The diagnosis can be made readily by an experienced observer, whether the biopsy comes from bone, spleen, or liver.

Gaucher[15] is usually credited with the first case report, under the title of "epithelioma of the spleen" (sic). Actually, our basic knowledge of the condition stems in large part from the pioneer pathologic studies of Brill, Mandelbaum, and Libman[7] and their successors[16-18] at Mount Sinai Hospital in New York. (Perhaps this explains why so many of the early case reports were in Jewish patients.)

Gaucher's disease is commonly encountered or recognized in adults and may pursue a chronic protracted course over a period of decades.[19] However, in recent years there have been a number of reports[9,10] of instances in infancy and early childhood featuring a more rapid course, so that the clinical differentiation from Niemann-Pick disease may be a problem. In this regard, the finding of Tuchman and his associates[17] that the serum acid phosphatase level is significantly elevated in Gaucher's disease may be helpful. There may be certain hematologic manifestations—specifically, hypochromic anemia, presumably from bone marrow encroachment, and leukopenia and thrombocytopenia (with a tendency to hemorrhage) from splenic involvement.

The osseous changes[8,18,20] are more relevant here. They may be demonstrable roentgenographically in many sites, but in general they are characterized by increased lucency, thinning of cortices, loss of cancellous bone markings, and sometimes expansion of the affected bone. Pathologic fracture may occasionally be observed. One of the best known changes, to which diagnostic importance is attached, is the tendency to cortical thinning and bilateral symmetrical flaring or fusiform expansion

Fig. 6-1. A, Skeletal changes in Gaucher's disease in a child. Note the cortical thinning and bilateral symmetrical flaring of the distal femur. **B,** Comparable changes in a humerus of the same patient. **C,** From another case of Gaucher's disease in a child, age 5, with involvement of upper femora, showing collapse of one and displacement of capital femoral epiphysis.

A   B

Fig. 6-2. A, Roentgenogram showing partial avascular necrosis (bone infarct) in the femoral head of an adult with Gaucher's disease. There are secondary osteoarthritic changes in the hip, but collapse of the head had not taken place (as it may). **B,** A bone infarct in the lower femoral shaft of the same patient. There was also a comparable old infarct in the opposite femur (not shown).

of the lower femora (Fig. 6-1, *A*). Comparable changes may be observed also in the distal humerus (Fig. 6-1, *B*). Involvement of vertebral bodies with collapse and resulting cord compression has been described, but this is unusual. Particular attention has also been directed to avascular necrosis in the femur, especially in the femoral head and neck, often followed by compression or collapse with subsequent osteoarthritic changes (Figs. 6-1, *C*, and 6-2, *A*).

There is not much that one can accomplish in the way of treatment beyond symptomatic relief, correction of anemia (if present), and appropriate orthopedic

management of such complications as infarction in a femoral head or compression of one or more vertebral bodies.

Irradiation of skeletal lesions, which enjoyed a brief vogue, is of questionable value and objectionable in principle. As for splenectomy, this should *not* be done casually, without very good indications, since removal of a major depot for lipid storage throws an added burden on the bone marrow and the liver, where the development of Gaucher's cirrhosis constitutes a serious problem.

Xanthoma tuberosum multiplex (lipid gout; essential hypercholesterolemia). Xanthoma tuberosum multiplex, a manifesta-

89

Fig. 6-3. Photomicrograph showing cholesterol deposition in tendinous tissue in xanthoma tuberosum multiplex.

tion of familial hyperlipoproteinemia, is characterized by hypercholesterolemia (up to 600 mg./100 ml.) and multiple cholesterol deposits in the skin, subcutis, and tendons, especially of the hands and feet, where pain and tumorous swelling may be produced.[21] This latter manifestation is well known to orthopedic surgeons. In present day biochemical parlance, it is encountered mainly with type II and occasionally with type III familial hyperlipoproteinemia, in which the levels of both cholesterol and triglyceride are elevated.[11] Occasionally there may be lipid storage in bone as well. I have seen a case in point in which there was resulting collapse of a vertebral body.

Examination of a representative specimen from the skin and subcutis or from a tumorous mass in a tendon shows abundant deposition and intermingling of cholesterol as crystals and also of cholesterol esters as foam cells (Fig. 6-3). As one might expect, the cholesterol crystals provoke foreign body reaction, but otherwise there is little or no inflammatory reaction.

One occasionally sees material from painful localized lesions in bone obtained as surgical specimens, which show cholesterol crystals and/or foam cells within fibrous connective tissue without any apparent basis for their deposition. As likely as not, such lesions are labeled "xanthoma" of bone for want of a more meaningful designation. I have seen a number of such puzzling instances, including several in an ulna and one in a scapula. In such cases, one should be circumspect about the possibility of familial hyperlipoproteinemia and check the serum cholesterol level, as well as the cutis and superficial tendons for possible lipid deposition.

Gout

The term "gout" has been used loosely in the past to refer to a number of conditions, including so-called calcium gout (calcinosis), lipid gout (xanthoma tuberosum multiplex), and even oxalic gout (oxalism). The present discussion deals exclusively with classical gout, which has plagued man since antiquity. It may be defined for basic orientation as a hereditary disorder of purine metabolism characterized by hyperuricemia, irregularly recurring attacks of acute arthritic involvement, and a tendency to urate deposition, often leading to more or less severe chronic tophaceous arthritis. The biochemical basis for these manifestations of sustained hyperuricemia is apparently quite complex,[22-26] and at least five forms of gout have been postulated,[25,26] with perhaps more to come.

Many persons (the relatives of gouty patients especially) may have a latent tendency to gout, manifested only by otherwise unexplained hyperuricemia, but they may never develop clinical gout. The latter is commonly ushered in by acute gout[27] affecting not only the first metatarsophalangeal joint (podagra) but frequently other joints as well. The incidence and severity of these sporadic, excruciatingly painful attacks vary considerably from case to case, and their pathogenetic basis has long been a matter of conjecture, although it was reported recently[28] that sodium urate crystals injected into the joints of volunteer gout patients caused a reaction very similar to an acute gout attack. In other words, acute gouty arthritis apparently represents microcrystalline synovitis,[25] but there is still much to be learned about this remarkable phenomenon. Between attacks (the so-called intercritical period), gouty patients may be ostensibly well, and many never develop significant tophaceous gout.[29] Some, however, after years of recurring episodes of acute gout, go on to develop chronic deforming changes associated with progressive urate deposition.[30] While this is ordinarily a relatively slow process, it may be remarkably accelerated at times.

It should also be noted that manifestations of gout may appear in patients with hematopoietic disorders in which the turnover of nucleic acids involved in hematopoiesis is accelerated, with excessive formation of uric acid. Whatever the reason for excessive urate formation, its accumulation is of potentially serious consequence in man (as distinct from lower mammalian species) because of enzymatic inability to convert uric acid to allantoin and because, normally, fully 80% of the glomerular urate filtrate is reabsorbed by the renal tubules. Moreover, the relatively low solubility of uric acid and its salts in tissue fluids also favors the insidious deposition of urate deposits in certain skeletal and extraskeletal sites of predilection, which will be indicated presently. It is essential to note further that in some gouty patients there is an associated tendency toward vascular disease of potentially serious import, reflected in a significantly high incidence of hypertension, severe nephrosclerosis with renal insufficiency, cardiac failure, and cerebrovascular accidents.[30]

Renewed interest has been evinced in gout in recent years, and from this clinical and biochemical research markedly improved therapeutic measures have evolved. One may cite here the proved effectiveness of phenylbutazone, corticotropin, and colchicine in terminating attacks of acute gout; the use of regular colchicine prophylaxis to reduce the incidence and severity of acute episodes; the administration of new uricosuric agents (such as probenecid, sulfinpyrazone, and allopurinol [HPP]) to help prevent chronic gouty arthritis and, with long-term good clinical control, to ameliorate established deformities and disability[31]; and the use of allopurinol (an inhibitor of uric acid synthesis), especially for gouty patients with a tendency to lithiasis.

That the skeletal connective tissues, particularly the joints and periarticular structures, bear the brunt of urate deposition in tophaceous gout is common knowledge. Within an affected joint (be it a metatarso-

Fig. 6-4. Low power photomicrograph showing the general appearance of urate deposits within bone. (×55.)

phalangeal, metacarpophalangeal, or interphalangeal joint, a knee, a hip, a shoulder, or any other), focal, chalky white or yellow, tophaceous deposits are observed on the articular surfaces. These deposits are also found in the deeper layers of the cartilage. The articular cartilage tends gradually to be destroyed and replaced by pannus (Fig. 15-10). Eventually, in severe instances with attendant deformity and immobilization, fibrous ankylosis may ensue, as well as the usual changes of secondary osteoarthritis. Concomitantly, the synovial lining and sublining connective tissue of the affected joint capsule likewise exhibit focal impregnation by urates. Eventually, more or less extensive reactive chronic villous synovitis ensues. The articular bone ends frequently manifest urate deposits within their periosteal covering, as well as in the subchondral spongy bone (Fig. 6-4). The ligaments and tendons, too, may be more or less heavily impregnated. Similarly, certain of the periarticular bursae, especially the olecranon and prepatellar bursae, are often predilected. In the vertebral column, the intervertebral disks and the contiguous portions of the bodies may be the sites of appreciable urate deposition.[30]

As for extraskeletal urate deposits, tophaceous involvement of the skin and subcutis, especially of the hands and feet and occasionally of the ear, is commonly observed in instances of moderate severity. Urate deposits are frequently encountered at necropsy in the kidney (where they favor the development of pyelonephritis), and occasionally in the lower urinary tract as stones or gravel. Involvement of the eye, of the heart and blood vessels, of the upper and lower airways, and of many other sites has been documented,[30] although today these are unusual, if not rare.

In chronic tophaceous gout, the charac-

Fig. 6-5. Photomicrograph of a representative field of a gouty tophus showing urate deposits characteristically ringed by foreign body giant cells, as well as smaller macrophages. This block was fixed in formalin rather than alcohol, and crystalline structure is lacking. (×250.)

teristic tissue response to urate deposits, wherever they may be encountered, is essentially that of a peculiar and distinctive foreign-body reaction (Fig. 6-5). The urate material usually appears rather amorphous in formalin-fixed specimens, and only in alcohol-fixed preparations does one regularly discern crystalline structure. On microscopic examination, one characteristically observes smaller or larger, discrete or conglomerate deposits, ringed peripherally by foreign body giant cells and/or mononuclear histiocytes. This reaction pattern is sufficiently distinctive for reliable diagnosis, and blackening with silver is scarcely required for confirmation. The inflammatory response otherwise is usually rather inconspicuous, provided that there has not been ulceration or complicating infection (which is unusual). At times, one may see calcification of urate deposits and even conspicuous heterotopic ossification.[30]

Hereditary ochronosis

Since Garrod[32] introduced the concept of inborn errors of metabolism in 1923, specific gene defects producing enzymatic abnormalities have been postulated for more than a hundred syndromes, and the list will undoubtedly continue to grow. Many of these disorders result from abnormal amino-acid metabolism. A substantial number may be responsible for mental retardation—phenylketonuria (PKU) is a well-known example. As with congenital disorders of skeletal development, it appears that everything that can possibly go wrong apparently does so at one time or another. The possibilities of error are so numerous that a whole cluster of diseases in point result from defects in the intermediary metabolism of phenylalanine and tyrosine alone—for example, phenylpyruvic oligophrenia, tyrosinosis, albinism, phenylketonuria, and hereditary ochronosis (alkaptonuria).

The present discussion will deal briefly with only one of these disorders, hereditary ochronosis,[33] which was selected because of its striking skeletal changes. For a comprehensive account of the genetic background and detailed pathologic changes, the reader may have recourse to my paper[34] on the subject published in 1954. Alkaptonuria reflects the urinary excretion of homogentisic acid (2, 5-dihydroxyphenylacetic acid) as one manifestation and usually the initial expression of hereditary ochronosis. As such, alkaptonuria is no more a disease per se than is glycosuria in relation to diabetes mellitus.

Far from being a harmless curiosity, as has often been implied, hereditary ochronosis results eventually in a more or less disabling arthritis and ankylosing spondylitis of a specific nature.[34-37] The development of calcific aortic stenosis may be another serious sequel. Still other deleterious effects of abnormal pigment deposition are severe arteriosclerosis, ochronotic nephrosis, and the formation of pigment calculi in the urinary tract.[34]

That the skeletal connective tissue structures bear the brunt of ochronotic pigment

Fig. 6-6. Roentgenogram of a segment of the lower lumbar vertebral column showing conspicuous radiopacity of the intervertebral disks. Also evident are the arthritic changes in the lumbosacral joint at the distal end of the specimen.

Fig. 6-7. Photograph (reduced) of a portion of the vertebral column (lower dorsal and lumbar) as viewed externally, showing blackened osteophytic rings at the levels of the intervertebral disks.

deposition is well known (Figs. 6-6 to 6-9). The bones themselves, apart from their articulations and their periosteal investment, are altered only to a limited extent. In affected synovial joints, the articular cartilage becomes hard, brittle, and pigmented and tends to break away piecemeal in the course of articular function, so that eventually the bone ends may be largely, if not entirely, denuded of cartilage (Fig. 15-11). When the involved joint is a comparatively large one, such as the knee, some of these pigmented cartilage fragments may constitute free joint bodies.[35] Many of them are ground into the synovium and the subsynovial connective tissue, producing the striking picture illustrated in Fig. 15-11, *B*. In these circumstances, it is not surprising that the synovium should show blackening and reactive villous synovitis or that, with continued function, marginal exostoses, conspicuous subchondral sclerosis, and other changes of secondary osteoarthritis of appreciable severity should ensue. While these changes of ochronotic arthritis develop slowly and usually become a clinical problem in middle age, pertinent cases have been recorded in which significant disability ensued long before the age of 40.

Equally important are the changes in the vertebral column; these lead eventually to a peculiar *ochronotic ankylosing spondylitis*. This has its basis in heavy impregnation of the intervertebral disks by ochronotic pigment, which is reflected roentgenographically by conspicuous radiopacity (Fig. 6-6). The pigment is deposited throughout the disks, in the anulus fibrosus, nucleus pulposus, and contiguous longitudinal ligament (where it provokes the formation of prominent, somewhat blackishly discolored, osteophytic rings; Fig. 6-7). The profoundly altered, impregnated disk tissue tends ultimately to be resorbed, and at many levels one may observe merely residual discontinuous remnants of it. The contiguous vertebral bodies manifest a tendency to fusion where the disk material is defective or absent (Fig. 6-8). The end result may be that of a substantially fused

Fig. 6-8. Photomicrograph of a section of the vertebral column showing an involved intervertebral disk. Most of the impregnated disk tissue has disappeared at this level and only discontinuous remnants of it are seen. Where the disk is defective, the contiguous vertebral bodies have fused.

Fig. 6-9. Photograph (reduced) showing conspicuous blackish discoloration of the costal cartilages and their perichondrium, as well as of the periosteum of the ribs and the intercostal ligaments.

"poker" spine showing abnormal curvature. In the light of these changes, one can readily appreciate the disability commonly associated with involvement of the vertebral column in ochronosis and the singularity of gait that Osler[38] described more than 60 years ago.

Brief mention may be made here to two other abnormalities of amino acid metabolism in which there are incidental skeletal effects. In *cystine storage disease* (cystinosis, Lignac-Fanconi disease), which shows many of the features of renal tubular transport disease (leakage of phosphate, glucose, amino acids, and so forth), characteristic crystals are deposited in the bone marrow, cornea, and reticulum-bearing tissues.

Also, in primary hyperoxaluria (*oxalism*), which is thought to reflect a defect or block in glycine metabolism, oxalate stones may form in the urinary tract and oxalate crystals may appear in the bone marrow, cartilage, kidney, heart muscle, and other sites. They show up as birefringent crystals when viewed with polarized light.

Porphyria

Porphyria results from an unusual inborn error of porphyrin metabolism, in which there is spontaneous excessive excretion of uroporphyrin and porphyrin precursors. The porphyrins in general are a remarkable group of pyrrole ring–containing, metal-binding, fluorescent chemical compounds found combined with protein in respiratory pigments, such as hemoglobin, cytochrome, and catalase. Another important member of the group is chlorophyll, a magnesium-porphyrin compound essential for photosynthesis in plants.

Despite the brilliant work of Hans Fischer on the chemical structure of the porphyrins over 50 years ago, we still know relatively little about their intermediary metabolism in man or about the precise nature of the enzymatic defect or aberration in human porphyria. The protean clinical manifestations of the disease, however, have been clarified, and it is now conventional[39,40] to classify cases of porphyria as falling into two types.

The first type, which constitutes a relatively small group, is *porphyria erythropoietica* (congenital), inherited as a mendelian recessive trait. It manifests itself in childhood by photosensitivity, increased hemolysis and increased erythropoiesis, red urine, reddish discoloration of teeth (*erythrodontia*), and staining also of the bone to a red or mahogany-brown. The last apparently reflects marked increase of marrow porphyrin within the growing bones. Fluorescent microscopy of such marrow samples shows intense red fluorescence concentrated in the nuclei of normoblasts.

The second type, which accounts for most of the clinical cases, is now designated at *porphyria hepatica.* It includes as subtypes *acute intermittent porphyria* and *porphyria cutanea tarda,* as well as occasional mixed forms and latent porphyria (most often found in relatives of patients with so-called hepatic porphyria). The most common expression of the disorder, acute intermittent porphyria, usually begins in early adult life and is characterized by potentially serious repeated crises, often with bizarre symptoms featuring abdominal pain (simulating that of an acute surgical abdomen), varied neurologic manifestations, and psychiatric disorders. In this expression of porphyria, as in the "cutanea tarda" form, excessive porphyrins or their precursors are said to be concentrated in the liver rather than the bone marrow, so that there are no noteworthy skeletal changes.

Systemic disorders of mucopolysaccharide metabolism

The best known skeletal disease caused by a mucopolysaccharide metabolic disorder is gargoylism, which was discussed in Chapter 2. Morquio's disease may well be another instance in point.

Another unusual storage disease that has some resemblance to gargoylism and that perhaps belongs here also has been described in several infants at autopsy by Farber, Cohen, and Uzman[41] under the title of "Lipogranulomatosis: a new lipo-glyco-protein storage disease." In this condition, as in gargoylism, the excessive abnormal storage material was found on chemical analysis to have a large polysaccharide residue (forming a complex with a polypeptide). Its anatomic distribution, however, apart from comparable central nervous system neuron involvement, was different. Specifically, in the cases cited there were widespread storage deposits within macrophages, predilecting the joints, the subcutaneous and periarticular tissues (featuring gout-like nodules, especially on the hands), the juxtaarticular bone, the larynx (hoarseness), the lymph nodes, and eventually the viscera, particularly the central nervous system and the lungs.

It seems likely that this category is still far from being completely delineated[42] and that, in time, still other comparable disorders may be recognized by astute observers. For detailed consideration of this group of inherited disorders, the reader should see the recent article by McKusick and his associates[43] on "The genetic mucopolysaccharidoses."

Some miscellaneous considerations

In long-standing, terminal cachectic states, one may commonly observe gelatinous atrophy of the fat cells in the bone marrow. For example, it is often possible to suspect that a patient died of carcinomatosis from examination of a section of the bone even before one learns of the clinical history.

In some long-standing infections, especially chronic osteomyelitis and tuberculosis, *amyloid* may be deposited in the parenchymatous organs, particularly the liver, spleen, adrenal glands, and kidneys. In contrast to this conventional pattern of distribution, one may occasionally find amyloid deposited in large quantities in bones, muscles, joint capsules, and skeletal connective tissues generally, as well as in the skin and subcutis, buccal and mucous membranes, tongue, heart, lungs, intestines, genitourinary tract, and other tissues. The basis for this atypical amyloidosis may be unsuspected multiple myeloma, but sometimes there is no apparent predisposing cause (idiopathic).

Influence of trace elements on the skeleton. As Asling and Hurley[44] have emphasized in their comprehensive survey of the various elements found in trace amounts in animal tissues, four elements—manganese, zinc, copper, and iodine—are clearly required for normal skeletal growth and development. A fifth, molybdenum, produces skeletal abnormalities when it is present in the diet in excess. Serious consequences to the epiphyseal cartilage plate may result from both manganese and zinc deficiencies, while copper deficiency appears to cause a defect in osseous replacement of cartilage. Moreover, in animals at least, manganese and zinc are required for normal elongation of the bones. As Asling points out further, in all of these deficiencies gross malformations of bone shape (especially in weight-bearing bones), of epiphyseal structure, or of joint relationships are reported frequently. The abnormalities may be recognized at several sites or may be more localized; this apparently varies with different species.[44-46]

The primary role of iodine is influencing activity of the thyroid gland, although it is also necessary for normal skeletal development.

Whether the abnormalities resulting from manganese, zinc, and copper deficiencies have their counterpart in humans, especially in young children, is a matter of conjecture. It is conceivable that they might in certain areas with mineral-deficient soils or under conditions of severe deprivation. However there are few, if any, relevant observations on which to base a judgment.

References

1. Sobotka, H., Epstein, E. Z., and Lichtenstein, L.: The distribution of lipoid in a case of Niemann-Pick's disease associated with amaurotic family idiocy, Arch. Path. **10**:677, 1930.
2. Crocker, A. C., and Farber, S.: Niemann-Pick disease, Medicine **37**:1, 1958; ibid., Amer. J. Clin. Nutr. **9**:63, 1961.
3. Lynn, R., and Terry, R. D.: Lipoid histochemistry and electron microscopy in adult Niemann-Pick disease, Amer. J. Med. **37**:987, 1964.
4. Terry, R. D., Sperry, W. M., and Brodoff, B.: Adult lipoidosis resembling Niemann-Pick's disease, Amer. J. Path. **30**:263, 1954.
5. Volk, B. W.: Tay-Sachs disease, New York, 1964, Grune and Stratton, Inc., pp. 36-67.
6. Volk, B. W., Adachi, M., Schneck, L., Saifer, A., and Kleinberg, W.: G$_5$—ganglioside variant of systemic late infantile lipoidosis, Arch. Path. **87**:393, 1969. (For recent literature.)
7. Brill, N. E., Mandelbaum, F. S., and Libman, E.: Primary splenomegaly, Gaucher type, Amer. J. Med. Sci. **129**:491, 1905.
8. Pick, L.: Die skelettform des Morbus Gaucher, Jena, 1927, Gustav Fisher Verlag.
9. Stein, M., and Gardner, L. I.: Acute infantile Gaucher's disease, Pediatrics **27**:491, 1961.
10. Harrison, W. E., Jr., and Louis, H. J.: Osseous Gaucher's disease in early childhood, J.A.M.A. **187**:997, 1964.
11. Wessler, S., and Avioli, L. A.: Classification and management of familial hyperlipoproteinemia, J.A.M.A. **207**:929, 1969.
12. Frederickson, D. S., Levy, R. I., and Lees, R. S.: Fat transport in lipoproteins—an integrated approach to mechanisms and disorders, New Eng. J. Med. **276**:34, 1967.
13. Rosenberg, A., and Chargoff, E.: Reinvestigation of cerebroside deposited in Gaucher's disease, J. Biol. Chem. **233**:1323, 1958.
14. Frederickson, D. S.: Cerebroside lipoidosis: Gaucher's disease. In Stanbury, J. B., Wynngarden, J. B., and Frederickson, D. S., editors: The metabolic basis of inherited disease, ed. 2, New York, 1966, McGraw-Hill Book Co., pp. 565-580.
15. Gaucher, P. C. E.: De l'epithéliome primitif de la rate, Thèse de Paris, 1882.
16. Arkin, A. M., and Schein, A. J.: Aseptic necrosis in Gaucher's disease, J. Bone Joint Surg. **30-A**:631, 1948.
17. Tuchman, L. R., Suna, H., and Carr., J. J.: Elevation of serum acid phosphatase in Gaucher's disease, J. Mount Sinai Hosp. N. Y. **23**:227, 1956.
18. Welt, S., Rosenthal, N., and Oppenheimer, B. S.: Gaucher's splenomegaly with special reference to skeletal changes, J.A.M.A. **92**:637, 1929.
19. Knox, J. H., Wahl, H. R., and Schmeisser, H. C.: Gaucher's disease, Bull. Johns Hopk. Hosp. **27**:1, 1916.
20. Milch, H., and Pomeranz, M.: Bone changes in Gaucher's splenomegaly, Ann. Surg. **89**:552, 1929.
21. Glueck, C. J., Levy, R. I., and Frederickson, D. S.: Acute tendinitis and arthritis: a presenting symptom of familial type II hyperlipoproteinemia, J.A.M.A. **206**:2895, 1968.
22. Editorial: Hyperuricemia and gout, Bull. Rheum. Dis. **18**:465, 1967.
23. Emerson, B. T.: An enzyme defect in metabolic gout, Ann. Intern. Med. **68**:707, 1968.

24. Gutman, A. B.: Some recent advances in the study of uric acid metabolism and gout: the musculoskeletal system: a symposium, presented at New York Academy of Medicine, October, 1950, New York, 1952, The Macmillan Co.

25. Editorial: Gout and hyperuricemia, Calif. Med. **110**:258, 1969.

26. Klinenberg, J. R.: Current concepts of hyperuricemia and gout, Calif. Med. **110**:231, 1969.

27. Sydenham, T.: A treatise on the gout (Tractatus de podagra et hydrope), London, 1683.

28. Medical news: Gout—no longer among the rheumatic aristocracy, J.A.M.A. **186**:40, 1963.

29. Talbott, J. H.: Gout and gouty arthritis, New York, 1953, Grune and Stratton, Inc.

30. Lichtenstein, L., Scott, H. W., and Levin, M. H.: Pathologic changes in gout: survey of eleven necropsied cases, Amer. J. Path. **32**:871, 1956.

31. Thompson, G. B., Duff, I. F., Robinson, W. L., Mikkelsen, W. M., and Galindez, H.: Long term uricosuric therapy in gout, Arthritis Rheum. **5**:384, 1962.

32. Garrod, A. E.: Inborn errors of metabolism, ed. 2, London, 1923, Hodder and Stoughton Ltd., pp. 43-64.

33. Virchow, R.: Ein fall von allgemeiner Ochronose der Knorpel und Knorpelähnlichen Teile, Virch. Arch. Path. Anat. **37**:212, 1866.

34. Lichtenstein, L., and Kaplan, L.: Hereditary ochronosis: pathologic changes observed in two necropsied cases, Amer. J. Path. **30**:99, 1954.

35. Sutro, C. J., and Anderson, M. E.: Alkaptonuric arthritis: cause for free intra-articular bodies, Surgery **22**:120, 1947.

36. La Du, B. N., Seegmiller, J. E., Laster, L., and Zannoni, V.: Alcaptonuria and ochronotic arthritis, Bull. Rheum. Dis. **8**:163, 1958.

37. O'Brien, W. M., Banfield, W. G., and Sokoloff, L.: Studies on the pathogenesis of ochronotic arthropathy, Arthritis Rheum. **4**:137, 1961.

38. Osler, W.: Ochronosis: the pigmentation of cartilages, sclerotics and skin in alkaptonuria, Lancet **1**:10, 1904.

39. Schwartz, S.: Clinical aspects of porphrin metabolism, Vet. Admin. Tech. Bull. TB10-94, December 1, 1953.

40. Seide, M. J.: Porphyria: report of nine cases diagnosed in the greater Hartford area, including a family with three affected, New Eng. J. Med. **258**:630, 1958.

41. Farber, S., Cohen, J., and Uzman, L. L.: Lipogranulomatosis: a new lipo-glyco-protein "storage" disease, J. Mount Sinai Hosp. N. Y. **24**:816, 1957.

42. Klenk, E.: The pathological chemistry of the developing brain. In Waelsch, H., editor: Biochemistry of the developing nervous system, New York, 1955, Academic Press, Inc., pp. 397-410.

43. McKusick, V. A., and others: The genetic mucopolysaccharidoses, Medicine **44**:445, 1965.

44. Asling, C. W., and Hurley, L. S.: The influence of trace elements on the skeleton, Clin. Orthop. **27**:213-264, 1963. (Extensive bibliography.)

45. Comar, C. L., and Bronner, F., editors: Mineral metabolism—an advanced treatise, vol. 2B, New York, 1962, Academic Press, Inc.

46. Underwood, E. J.: Trace elements in human and animal nutrition, New York, 1956, Academic Press, Inc.

General references

Galdston, M., Steele, J. M., and Dobiner, K.: Alkaptonuria and ochronosis, with a report of three patients and metabolic studies in two, Amer. J. Med. **13**:432, 1952.

Stanbury, J. B., Wynngarden, J. B., and Frederickson, D. S.: The metabolic disease of inherited disease, ed. 2, New York, 1966, McGraw-Hill Book Co.

Chapter 7

Skeletal changes in renal disease

Some 30 years ago, Rutishauser and his associates,[1] Ginzler and Jaffe,[2] and other investigators showed that in cases of protracted renal insufficiency in adults (resulting from chronic glomerulonephritis, pyelonephritis, hydronephrosis, or pyonephrosis), one can consistently find *resorptive skeletal changes.* Such patients clinically manifest azotemia, phosphate retention, depressed serum calcium level, and lowered carbon dioxide–combining power, reflecting acidosis. Although the bones may appear normal grossly at the time of autopsy, the spongy trabeculae, especially of vertebral bodies, are likely to show at least occasional resorption lacunae on their surface. These lacunae are usually filled with connective tissue and possibly a few osteoclasts (Fig. 7-1).

When the changes are more advanced, these resorption tracts are more prominent and may also involve the cortical bone around the haversian canals. At the same time, reparative new bone apposition may be evident; this is usually slight, but occasionally it may overshadow the resorptive changes so that the end result can be a closely compacted spongiosa or "renal osteosclerosis."[2] In such cases, the parathyroid glands usually show slight to moderate enlargement with chief cell hyperplasia, or only microscopic hyperplasia without obvious enlargement of the glands. However, Ginzler and Jaffe felt, as had Rutishauser,

that there was no compelling reason to invoke a factor of functional secondary hyperparathyroidism. They believed rather that the osseous changes noted could be plausibly explained on the basis of *chronic acidosis* induced by the renal insufficiency.

To be sure, as many investigators have pointed out,[3-7] there are other instances of chronic renal insufficiency in which the parathyroid glands are distinctly enlarged and in which there is convincing clinical, biochemical, and roentgenographic evidence of *secondary hyperparathyroidism.* In fact, it should be emphasized that chronic renal insufficiency is by far the most common cause of secondary hyperparathyroidism. The latter, in turn, may cause renal damage from nephrocalcinosis. A good history of primary renal disease may be necessary to unravel the complex picture that eventually ensues.

As previously indicated (Chapter 4), when secondary hyperparathyroidism complicating renal insufficiency develops in a growing patient, osseous changes clinically and pathologically resembling those of infantile vitamin D–deficiency rickets may develop (Fig. 7-2). In the older literature, such cases were called "renal rickets,"[8] although this designation is no longer in favor ("renal osteodystrophy" is preferred). As a rule, the condition manifests itself in older children (7 to 12 years of age is the usual range) and is associated with a tendency

Fig. 7-1. Photomicrograph showing skeletal resorptive changes associated with long-standing, chronic renal insufficiency.

Fig. 7-2. Roentgenograms showing the changes of so-called renal rickets in the femur and lower tibia.

to dwarfism and infantilism. Later in the course of the disease or terminally, one may sometimes see calcific deposits in the arteries, in the soft tissues near the joints, and in the skin and subcutaneous tissue. The underlying renal disorder is likely to be some congenital defect, such as hydronephrosis, hypogenesis, or some obstructive malformation with secondary infection. In these circumstances, therapy usually has distinct limitations.

It appears also that there are occasional cases of secondary hyperparathyroidism complicating protracted renal insufficiency (from glomerulonephritis) in older patients beyond the growth period. In such cases the skeletal changes are said to resemble those of osteomalacia. Such instances have been designated *renal osteomalacia*. They must be unusual, however; I have not had occasion to examine at first hand any material from a case in point as a basis for independent judgment.

Following repeated hemodialysis for chronic renal failure, a striking increase in skeletal complications (from about 25% to 80% or more) has been noted, despite control of the uremia. Florid renal osteodystrophy and soft-tissue calcification have become important life-threatening complications of therapy by mechanical means. Concomitantly, it has been observed after renal transplantation that hyperparathyroidism may be protracted long after renal failure has been overcome (tertiary or autonomous hyperparathyroidism). These serious problems, along with disordered divalent iron metabolism, are currently under active clinical investigation.

As previously indicated (Chapter 4), when osteomalacia (or rickets, for that matter) develops from a renal disorder, the latter is much more likely to be in the nature of a defect of tubular reabsorption in which the kidneys leak excessive amounts of phosphate, glucose, certain amino acids, or possibly other metabolites (*Debré-de Toni-Fanconi syndrome*).[9] This inability of the proximal convoluted tubules to reabsorb essential components of the glomerular filtrate may result from a number of noxious chemical agents—such as copper (as in Wilson's disease) and lead, among others—or from such conditions as myeloma and sarcoidosis. However, it more often reflects a congenital, sometimes familial, enzymatic defect. The significant persistent loss of phosphate in an affected child leads to rachitic changes requiring very large, if not massive, doses of vitamin D for effective control (so-called metabolic rickets or hypophosphatemic vitamin D–resistant rickets). In these circumstances, stunting of stature, reflecting short lower limb bones, and bowing deformities often requiring surgical correction are commonly observed.[10]

In some cases in point, there is *glycosuria* as well (so-called renal diabetes), but this can be readily overcome. More serious manifestations may result from concomitant *aminoaciduria*, notably cirrhosis of the liver with hepatic insufficiency, the pathogenesis of which is not clear. Certain amino acids in particular have been implicated, especially cystine and glycine. Specifically, it appears[11] that in cystine storage disease, tubular reabsorption may be impaired and that there may eventually be failure of renal excretory function. Glycine leakage in the urine has also been described[12] as an unusual cause of muscle weakness associated with osteomalacic skeletal changes (in somewhat older children or young adults). Mental retardation and glaucoma are still other unusual complications of tubule reabsorption disease that have been noted.[13]

Apparently there can be many possible factors in varying combination in this disorder, and any attempt at this time to classify them beyond a very provisional working hypothesis seems premature. Inasmuch as available clinical material for further investigation is limited, it may be quite a while before the entire picture is elucidated.

References

1. Rutishauser, E.: Ostéodystrophie nephrogène, Ann. Anat. Path. **13**:999, 1936.
2. Ginzler, A. M., and Jaffe, H. L.: Osseous findings in chronic renal insufficiency in adults, Amer. J. Path. **17**:293, 1941.
3. Albright, F., Drake, T. G., and Sulkowitch, H. W.: Renal osteitis fibrosa cystica; review of a case with discussion of metabolic aspects, Bull. Johns Hopk. Hosp. **60**:377, 1937.
4. Carnot, P., and Lafitte, A.: Chronic nephritis, hyperparathyroidism and skeletal changes, J.A.M.A. **110**:1683, 1938.
5. Castleman, B., and Mallory, T. B.: Parathyroid hyperplasia in chronic renal insufficiency, Amer. J. Path. **13**:553, 1937.
6. Highman, W. J., Jr., and Hamilton, B.: Hyperparathyroidism in kidney disease, J. Clin. Invest. **16**:103, 1937.
7. Pappenheimer, A. M., and Wilens, S. L.: Enlargement of the parathyroid glands in renal disease, Amer. J. Path. **11**:73, 1935.
8. Shelling, D. H., and Remsen, D.: Renal rickets: report of a case showing four enlarged parathyroids and evidence of parathyroid hypersecretion, Bull. Johns Hopk. Hosp. **57**:158, 1935.
9. De Toni, G.: Renal rickets with phospho-gluco-amino renal diabetes (de Toni-Debré-Fanconi syndrome), Ann. Pediat. **16**:479, 1933; ibid. **187**:42, 1956.
10. Tapia, J., Stearns, G., and Ponseti, I. V.: Vitamin D resistant rickets: a long-term clinical study of 11 patients, J. Bone Joint Surg. **46-A**: 935, 1964.
11. Worthin, H., and Good, R.: J. Dis. Child. **95**:653, 1958.
12. Dent, C. E., and Harris, H. J.: Hereditary forms of rickets and osteomalacia, J. Bone Joint Surg. **38**:204, 1956.
13. Lowe, C. U., Terry, M., and MacLachlan, E. A.: Organic-aciduria, decreased renal ammonia production, hydrophthalmas, and mental retardation; clinical entity, Amer. J. Dis. Child. **83**:164, 1952.

General references

Dent, C. E.: Aminoaciduria in Fanconi syndrome, Biochem. J. **41**:240, 1947.
Fraser, D.: Clinical manifestations of genetic aberrations of calcium and phosphorus metabolism, J.A.M.A. **176**:113, 1961.
Fraser, D., and Salter, R. B.: Pediat. Clin. N. Amer. **5**:417, 1958.

Chapter 8

Osteoporosis (osteopenia)

Osteoporosis, in which there is *too little bone* for a variety of reasons, is probably the most common of all the metabolic bone disorders. More specifically, osteoporotic bone has fewer and thinner trabeculae. This is not the result of vascular or osteoclastic resorption but rather of decreased bone formation and, sometimes, excessive bone breakdown with increased urinary excretion of bone-forming minerals.[1] The serum calcium, phosphorus, and alkaline phosphatase levels are ordinarily within the normal range.

The most common causes of osteoporosis fall into three major categories: (1) disuse atrophy from immobilization, (2) diminution or loss of anabolic sex hormones, especially in women 10 years or more past spontaneous menopause, but also in eunuchoid states, senility, and gonadal dysgenesis (Turner's syndrome), and (3) excess of catabolic hormones, specifically in thyrotoxicosis[2] or in Cushing's syndrome, occurring either spontaneously (which is unusual) or, more often, after the therapeutic administration of large doses of cortisone or other corticoids. As Gordan[12] has emphasized, all the available corticoids rapidly produce calcium wasting and can cause clinical osteoporosis (Fig. 8-1). In cases of spontaneous Cushing's disease coming to autopsy, the bones become so soft and thin that one can cut them with a knife, without decalcification.

Still other, relatively infrequent causes of osteoporosis are long-standing malnutrition, gastrectomy, pregnancy[3] (particularly in the last trimester), acromegaly, biliary cirrhosis,[4] and scurvy. In some of these conditions, the mechanism of bone loss is not as well understood as it might be. When the cause of osteoporosis cannot be pinpointed, it is called "idiopathic," but the number of such cases has apparently dwindled in recent years. Some of these respond to intravenous administration of serum albumin.[5]

Osteoporosis usually involves the weight-bearing vertebrae primarily; quite understandably, pain in the lumbar spine is a common presenting complaint. In the common postmenopausal type of osteoporosis this may be the only significant skeletal alteration.[6-9] In milder grades of osteoporosis, it is important to establish that the apparent loss of bone observed radiographically is genuine, rather than the reflection of various technical factors. This is easier said than done, however, for radiologists have experienced difficulty in establishing consistently reliable criteria for the determination of early osteopenia. It is only when the condition is far advanced or severe, as in Cushing's syndrome[10] or hyperparathyroidism,[5] that one sees comparable changes in the skull, ribs, and long bones.

In the vertebral column, the earliest roentgenographic changes are found in the

Fig. 8-1. Photograph showing severe osteoporosis of vertebral bodies developing after the therapeutic administration of large doses of steroids.

lower thoracic and lumbar vertebrae. As the spongy trabeculae become progressively sparse and delicate, the cortical rims stand out by contrast. Also, as the vertebral bodies are weakened they become biconcave, and the intervertebral disks expand accordingly (Figs. 8-2 and 8-3). In these circumstances, wedge fractures (often without injury) are common, and there is likewise a tendency to kyphosis and loss of stature. Another potentially serious complication is nephrolithiasis from hypercalcuria. One should therefore be wary of administering calcium and vitamin D for osteoporosis.

The roentgenographic changes indicated previously are, of course, not specific for osteoporosis. It is incumbent upon the observer to rule out the possibility of metastatic carcinomatosis (particularly from the breast) and of advanced multiple myeloma, which can produce comparable changes, as well as localized rarefying disorders of the spine other than osteoporosis, which can simulate such changes.

In the matter of clinical management, one must again stress the necessity for exclusion of other causes of rarefying bone disease, especially in the vertebral column, as well as recognition of the specific cause of osteoporosis and its correction, if possible. Adrenal cortical tumors can be removed, and thyrotoxicosis, immobilization, or malnutrition can be corrected. As Gordan and his associates[12,13] have emphasized, the most important single cause that can be treated effectively is hormonal deficiency in the postmenopausal or hypogonadal patient. For this they have used cyclically administered oral estrogens for their anabolic effect to great advantage, and without inducing carcinoma in a single

105

Diseases of bone and joints

Fig. 8-2. Roentgenogram showing thinning of vertebrae (dorsal and lumbar) and expansion of intervertebral disks. Osteoporosis developed spontaneously for no apparent cause.

Fig. 8-3. Photograph of sagittal section of lower dorsal and lumbar vertebral column of a woman past 70, showing the changes of advanced osteoporosis.

instance. Estrogen therapy provides positive calcium balance and stops bone destruction,[13] so that the tendency to fractures and loss of height is controlled; it does not, however, induce skeletal remineralization.[12]

References

1. Eisenberg, E., and Gordan, G. S.: Skeletal dynamics in man measured by nonradioactive strontium, J. Clin. Invest. **40:**1809, 1961.
2. Williams, R. H., and Morgan, H. J.: Thyrotoxic osteoporosis, Int. Clin. **2:**48, 1940.
3. Nordin, B. E. C., and Roper, A.: Post-pregnancy osteoporosis: a syndrome? Lancet **1:**431, 1955.
4. Atkinson, M., Nordin, B. E. C., and Sherlock, S.: Malabsorption and bone disease in prolonged obstructive jaundice, Quart. J. Med. **25:**299, 1956.
5. Albright, F., and Reifenstein, E. C., Jr.: The parathyroid glands and metabolic bone disease, Baltimore, 1948, Williams & Wilkins Co.
6. Gershon-Cohen, J., Rechtman, A. M., Schraer, H., and Blumberg, N.: Asymptomatic fractures in osteoporotic spines of the aged, J.A.M.A. **153:**625, 1953.
7. Kelly, M., Little, K., and Courts, A.: Bone matrix and osteoporosis, Lancet **1:**1125, 1959.
8. Schmorl, G., and Junghanns, H.: Die Gesunde und die Kranke Wirbelsaüle in Röntgenbild und Klinik, ed. 4, Stuttgart, 1957, Georg Thieme Verlag, pp. 71-81.
9. Urist, M.: Observations bearing on the prob-

lem of osteoporosis. In Rodahl, K., Nicholson, J., and Brown, M., Jr., editors: Bone as a tissue, New York, 1960, McGraw-Hill Book Co., p. 18.

10. Howland, W. J., Pugh, D. G., Jr., and Sprague, R. G.: Roentgenologic changes of the skeletal system in Cushing's syndrome, Radiology 71:69, 1958.

11. Solomon, G. F., Dickerson, W. J., and Eisen-

berg, E.: Psychologic and osteometabolic responses to sex hormones in elderly osteoporotic women, Geriatrics 15:46, 1960.

12. Gordan, G. S.: Osteoporosis: diagnosis and treatment, Texas State J. Med. 57:740, 1961.

13. Gordan, G. S., and Eisenberg, E.: The effect of estrogens, androgens and corticoids on skeletal kinetics in man, Proc. Roy. Soc. Med. 56:1027, 1963.

Chapter 9

Skeletal changes in neurotrophic disorders

The major neurotrophic disorders associated with spinal cord disease are Charcot neuroarthropathy from tabes dorsalis, which mainly affects the joints of the lower extremity and the spine, and comparable changes in the upper extremity from syringomyelia. The concept of joint destruction as a neurotrophic manifestation dates back fully a century to the observations of the brilliant French neurologist, Charcot.[1]

There are many other conditions, however, that should be cited here. On occasion, destructive neurotrophic changes in the foot may be observed in neglected or poorly controlled diabetes mellitus of long standing (Fig. 9-1). This subject has received considerable attention in recent years, and an awareness of it is important because the process can often be halted or even substantially improved by adequate diabetic treatment and corrective orthopedic measures.[2-4] Also noteworthy is the observation that spinal cord damage associated with spina bifida or severe multiple sclerosis, or resulting from cord injury with irreparable paraplegia,[5] may predispose to parosteal ossification, particularly in the vicinity of the hip and knee joints (Fig. 9-2).

Neuroarthropathy has also been said to be a sequel of injury to peripheral nerves (from trauma or tumor compression); for example, neuroarthropathy of an ankle joint may result from severance of the sciatic nerve,[6] although this is distinctly unusual. The classical example of extensive neurotrophic changes resulting from peripheral nerve disease is the neural form of leprosy in which there may be loss of digits and other mutilating deformities of the hands and/or feet, especially in patients whose disease is not controlled by sulfone therapy (Fig. 9-3). For a comprehensive list of still other unusual or rare causes of neuropathies of bones and joints (and the responsible disease foci may be in the brain, spinal cord, or peripheral nerves), the reader may have recourse to the old article of Shands,[7] which is still useful for orientation (Fig. 9-4).

By far the most common cause of neuroarthropathy is *tabes dorsalis*[8] (old-fashioned locomotor ataxia), an expression of untreated syphilis that has resulted in sclerosis of the posterior or dorsal columns of the spinal cord. The knee joint is commonly involved in this condition (Fig. 9-5), although the hip joints and the vertebral column may also be affected (Fig. 9-6). Only occasionally does one observe comparable involvement of a joint in the upper

Fig. 9-1. Roentgenogram of a neurotrophic foot in a diabetic patient who also had a long-standing, refractory trophic ulcer.

extremity, such as an elbow (Fig. 9-7). While Charcot joints are usually painless, there are enough exceptions to this rule so that the diagnosis cannot be dismissed because of the presence of pain.

There has been much speculation in the past about the pathogenesis of the striking destructive changes in a Charcot joint. In my opinion, what apparently happens is that, with loss of proprioceptive muscle sense resulting from dorsal column disease, there is malalignment of the bone ends of the affected joint in the course of articular function. The repeated trauma, in time, results in multiple osteoarticular fractures with breaking off of numerous fragments, some of which float as joint bodies, while others are ground into the joint capsule (Fig. 9-8). Each of the osseous fragments embedded within or deep to the synovium acts as a nidus around which new bone may be formed. As a result, the synovium becomes thickened and chronically inflamed, while the joint capsule as a whole

Fig. 9-2. Metaplastic ossification contiguous to the upper shaft of a femur in a case of multiple sclerosis with extensive severe spinal cord damage. (Comparable lesions are observed more often in paraplegic patients.)

109

Fig. 9-3. Photograph (reduced) showing mutilating changes in the hands in the neural form of leprosy.

Fig. 9-4. Roentgenogram of an amputated foot showing advanced neurotrophic changes caused by a spinal cord defect (possibly congenital, although not spina bifida). The metatarsal bones have disappeared, and there is atrophy of the remaining phalanges.

Fig. 9-5. Roentgenograms showing two Charcot knee joints in an advanced stage.

A   B

Fig. 9-6. A, Another patient with bilateral Charcot hips and also a Charcot spine (lumbar). B, Roentgenogram showing another Charcot spine.

111

Fig. 9-7. Roentgenogram of an unusual Charcot elbow joint in a man of 58 with tabes dorsalis. At autopsy, evidence of cardiovascular syphilis was also found.

Fig. 9-8. Photomicrograph (at low magnification) showing the characteristic changes in the synovial lining of a Charcot knee. Note the numerous fragments of articular cartilage and bone detritus ground into the membrane, which is thickened and chronically inflamed.

Fig. 9-9. **A,** Roentgenogram showing neuroarthropathy of a shoulder joint in a patient with syringomyelia. **B,** Neuroarthropathy at the wrist of another patient with syringomyelia.

tends to become distended, boggy, and fluid-filled. Eventually, marked destruction, deformity, and luxation of the articular bone ends ensues (Figs. 9-5 to 9-7). In the process of traumatic damage to articular cartilage, extensive changes of secondary osteoarthritis inevitably develop. This, of course, is a prominent feature of the fully developed lesion.

Another important though far less frequent cause of neuroarthropathy, especially in the upper extremity, is *syringomyelia* (syrinx of the spinal cord at the cervical level). This too is an old observation,[7] dating back about 80 years. It is estimated[9] that in some 25% of cases of syringomyelia, changes comparable to those described may develop in the shoulder, elbow, or wrist joints (Fig. 9-9). On occasion there may be trophic changes in the hand as well (Fig. 9-10).

Fig. 9-10. Roentgenogram showing trophic changes in the hand in syringomyelia.

113

References

1. Charcot, J. M.: Sur quelques arthropathies qui paraissent d'ependre d'une lésion du cerveau ou de la moelle épinière, Arch. Physiol. Norm. Path. 1:161, 1868.
2. Bailey, C. C., and Root, H. F.: Neuropathic foot lesions in diabetes mellitus, New Eng. J. Med. 236:397, 1947.
3. Martin, M. M.: Charcot joints in diabetes mellitus, Proc. Roy. Soc. Med. 45:503, 1952.
4. Degenhardt, D. P., and Goodwin, M. A.: Neuropathic joints in diabetics, J. Bone Joint Surg. 42-B:769, 1960.
5. Liberson, M.: Soft tissue calcifications in cord lesions, J.A.M.A. 152:1010, 1953.
6. Kerwein, G., and Lyons, W. F.: Neuroarthropathy of the ankle joint from complete severence of the sciatic nerve, Ann. Surg. 115:267, 1942.
7. Shands, A. R.: Neuropathies of the bones and joints, Arch. Surg. 20:614, 1930.
8. Steindler, A., Williams, L. A., and Puig, J.: Tabetic arthropathies, Urol. Cut. Rev. 46:633, 1942.
9. Luck, J. V.: Bone and joint diseases, Springfield, Illinois, 1950, Charles C Thomas, Publisher, p. 255.

Chapter 10

Skeletal changes in certain blood diseases

This section will deal primarily with a number of blood disorders in which the skeletal alterations are noteworthy or important. These disorders are, specifically, hemophilia (and other coagulation deficiency diseases producing comparable effects) and the chronic hemolytic anemias, particularly sickle cell anemia, thalassemia major, and spherocytic anemia. For a comprehensive discussion of these conditions and an appreciation of this rapidly developing frontier in molecular biology and genetics, the reader may have recourse to the last edition of the encyclopedic monograph of Wintrobe.[1] For more detailed consideration of the roentgenographic changes that may be observed, the text of Caffey[2] is valuable for orientation.

To avoid repetition, only brief mention is made here of myelosclerosis, mastocytosis, multiple myeloma, and the skeletal manifestations of malignant lymphoma, since these conditions have been discussed in my book, *Bone Tumors*.[3]

Hemophilia

Hemophilia has been known since ancient times as a congenital disease of bleeders. In modern genetic parlance, it results from the hereditary transmission of a sex-linked recessive mendelian trait to affected males. The frequency of hemophilic male births has been estimated[4] to be about one in 10,000, so the condition is by no means rare.

Hematologic research has shown that there are several types of hemophilia. In classical type A, blood clotting factor VIII (platelet cofactor [AHF]) is either not present in adequate concentration or is inhibited. There are all grades of clinical severity, depending on the blood level of factor VIII. In hemophilia B, or Christmas disease, there is a deficiency of factor IX (plasma thromboplastin component [PTC]). Other conditions resembling hemophilia and presenting essentially the same clinical manifestations result from deficiency of still other components involved in blood clotting (plasma thromboplastin antecedent [PTA], factor XII, and so on) or from the action of certain anticoagulants.[1,5]

However one pinpoints the coagulation deficiency in any given instance (and this is still an active area of investigation),[6] the tendency to prolonged and excessive bleeding usually appears in early childhood and may lead to repeated episodes of hemorrhage into skin and mucous membranes, muscles, eyes, various internal sites, bones, and joints. More than half of all hemophiliacs bleed into their joints.[7] The knee

115

Fig. 10-1. Roentgenogram showing changes in the knee joint in a child with hemophilia—specifically, thickening of the joint capsule, narrowing of the joint space (reflecting erosion of articular cartilage), irregularity of the articular bone ends (presumably from secondary osteoarthritis), and the presence of lucent defects within the epiphyseal bone (suggesting intramedullary hemorrhage).

is most often involved (Fig. 10-1), although the hip, ankle, elbow, and other joints may be affected.[8] Rapidly developing hemarthrosis in hemophilia is likely to be painful and disabling, presumably from increased intraarticular pressure and distension of the joint capsule. Initially, the blood is resorbed, but repeated (untreated) episodes over a period of years can lead to irreparable joint damage.[9]

In small joints, substantial osteoarticular destruction may result. In a large joint like the knee, more or less pronounced capsular swelling ensues from villous hypertrophy and fibrous thickening. Eventually the synovial lining becomes a deep forest-like web

or tangled mat of brownishly discolored villi. Its gross appearance may resemble that seen in diffuse pigmented villonodular synovitis, although (histiocytic) nodules are lacking. In time, the articular cartilage may be overgrown and eroded; then, of course, the changes of secondary osteoarthritis come into play. In a late stage, muscle atrophy, contracture, fibrous ankylosis, and permanent deformity may be sequelae of chronic, long-standing hemarthrosis.

The potential long-term seriousness of these manifestations underscores the importance of prevention. For control of bleeding, the prompt administration of factor VIII in sufficient amount to achieve a hemostatic level (a concentration of 25% or more of estimated normal) is indicated.[1] Type-specific whole blood or plasma may be used, but fresh frozen plasma is preferable, and high-potency antihemophilic factor (AHF) concentrate is now also available.[10] Under this protective cover repeated aspiration of blood from a joint and even surgery can be performed safely,[11] as required.

At times, hemorrhage in bone or its periosteum, apart from joint involvement, may also have serious consequences for hemophiliacs if it is not controlled or well managed, although this is encountered less often. It is usually the shaft of a large limb bone, notably the femur or the tibia, that is the site of massive hemorrhage, but other bones may also be affected. Frequently there is a large hematoma in muscle as well. Extensive hemorrhage within or beneath the periosteum is followed by organization and periosteal new bone formation, much as it is in scurvy. It appears from published reports[8] that in old neglected cases there may also be more or less extensive ragged or moth-eaten erosion of the bone cortex. In such circumstances there is a great hazard of pathologic fracture. Radiographically discernible, intramedullary hemorrhage may likewise be a prominent feature. Altogether, it is not surprising that such patients are sometimes operated on for suspected malignant tumor (the diagnosis is later changed to "pseudotumor"). In the old days, without adequate preparation or treatment, not a few succumbed to fatal hemorrhage or infection.

Chronic hemolytic anemias

In the chronic hemolytic anemias, as Caffey[2] has emphasized, the skeletal changes, in children at least, may be pathognomonic and often are among the most characteristic features. As indicated, the major conditions in point are sickle cell anemia, thalassemia, and spherocytic anemia. All of them are transmitted as mendelian traits and appear in a major, clinically significant form when homozygous. In each of them, the defect or abnormality in the red blood cells responsible for increased hemolysis, anemia, and sometimes icterus is specific and unique, as will be indicated presently. In general, however, this may be said with a view to understanding better the bone changes in all of them. In response to increased destruction of erythrocytes, the bone marrow becomes markedly hyperplastic. Within expansile, young growing bones, the marrow overgrowth causes widening of their medullary cavities and pressure atrophy of cortical and spongy bone, reflected radiographically in certain distinctive patterns. To be sure, the relative incidence, extent, and distribution of these skeletal alterations are variable.

Sickle cell anemia. In sickle cell disease (sicklemia), the red blood cells tend to assume a sickle (or oat) shape when oxygen pressure is reduced. The disease is caused by a dominant allele that occurs in variable frequencies, as high as 28% in different African Negro races[4] and about 8% in American Negroes. Sicklemia or sickle cell trait may produce few, if any, clinical manifestations. However, a small percentage of individuals with this disease (about

one in forty) develops potentially serious, hemolytic, sickle cell anemia.[12]

It was in connection with sickle cell anemia that the search for abnormal hemoglobins was started by Pauling[12] and his associates some 20 years ago. This is still an active field of investigation. More than eighty abnormal hemoglobins have now been identified,[1] with more undoubtedly on the way. Apparently, every alteration in the polypeptide chain structure gives rise to another addition to the wide range of abnormal hemoglobins.

Sickle cell anemia is characterized clinically by symptoms of anemia, arthritic manifestations (aching in the joints or elsewhere in the extremities, often ascribed to "rheumatism"), chronic leg ulcers (common in adolescents and adults, especially over the malleoli), and acute attacks of pain (abdominal cramps). As previously noted, bone infarcts may develop, especially in the capital femoral epiphysis (often with residual joint damage), the hand and foot bones, and even vertebral bodies (leading to compression). Curiously enough, osteomyelitis due to *Salmonella* appears to be a special hazard (Fig. 10-2, *A*).

In response to the hemolytic anemia, the bone marrow undergoes compensatory hyperplasia. As many as 50% to 70% of the nucleated cells may be nucleated red cells. On the whole, however, as contrasted with thalassemia, marrow hyperplasia is less pronounced, bone changes are less constant, symptoms often appear at a later age, and even severely affected patients survive longer.

When osseous changes occur in childhood (and they are often absent), one may observe involvement of metacarpals and proximal phalanges (so-called sickle cell dactylitis) or of the corresponding foot bones. If the long limb bones are affected, these may show cortical thinning and widening (Fig. 10-2, *B*). Sometimes the only demonstrable alterations may be in the

Fig. 10-2. A, Roentgenogram of a child with sickle cell anemia showing widening of the bones, especially of the metacarpals and proximal phalanges, and thinning of their cortices. The loss of the middle and distal phalanges of the third finger was a sequel of *Salmonella* osteomyelitis. **B,** From the case illustrated in **A,** showing cortical thinning and flaring (from marrow hyperplasia) in the distal metaphysis of the femur.

skull bones, especially the parietal and frontal bones; on occasion, the nasal, facial, and jaw bones may also be involved. The essential changes in the calvarium are thickening from widening of the diploë, as well as the formation of spicules of new bone, oriented perpendicularly to the inner table. Bone deformities such as kyphosis, scoliosis, saber shins, and oxycephaly are also observed at times, though not as often as in thalassemia. In adults, one may find evidence of previous bone infarcts, hemorrhage and fibrosis of the marrow, patchy osteosclerosis, and endosteal bone apposition, so that the cortices of large limb bones may actually be thickened.

Thalassemia. Thalassemia major (from the Greek word *thalassa* meaning sea), also designated in the older literature as Cooley's erythroblastic anemia and Mediterranean anemia, is caused by a specific, recessive allele that occurs in low frequency in various Mediterranean groups (it appears to be absent in central and northern European populations). Accordingly, the condition is largely confined either to people living on the Mediterranean shores, mainly Greeks, Italians, Syrians, and Armenians, or to their descendants, wherever they may be. In these groups, the frequency of carriers of the thalassemia trait has been estimated[4] at about one in twenty-five persons.

Like sickle cell anemia, thalassemia represents a molecular disease of abnormal hemoglobin. Recent hematologic research[13] has indicated that there are several genetic subtypes of thalassemia, featuring the pres-

118

Fig. 10-3. A, Roentgenogram of the skull of a child with thalassemia major (Cooley's anemia) showing pronounced thickening of the anterior portion of the calvarium and, in the parietal area particularly, striae of new bone oriented perpendicularly to the outer table. **B,** The hand bones in the same case as **A,** illustrating uniform cortical thinning of the metacarpals and phalanges and peculiar alteration of their spongy bone architecture. The metacarpal bones in particular have a rectangular contour in their projection (see also Fig. 10-4, *B*).

ence of significantly increased amounts in erythrocytes of fetal hemoglobin and/or hemoglobin A_2.

The clinical (homozygous) disease state (thalassemia major) may be manifested as early as the first year of life, is usually progressive in the growing child, and in severe cases may terminate fatally before adolescence. It is characterized by persistent anemia (responding temporarily to transfusions), icterus (reflecting elevated serum bilirubin from increased destruction of erythrocytes), elevated serum iron, hepatosplenomegaly, and certain bone changes (whose roentgenographic appearance is of diagnostic value). The bone marrow is hyperplastic and contains many immature

forms, including numerous normoblasts and megaloblasts. It also contains hemosiderin-laden macrophages and foam cells as a sequel of erythrocytic destruction.

The striking skeletal changes in the skull, long bones, hand bones, vertebral column, and other sites have already been mentioned (p. 117). Some of the more distinctive alterations are illustrated in Figs. 10-3 and 10-4 and are highlighted in the accompanying legends. It should be noted also that associated skeletal developmental anomalies are not infrequent and that premature fusion of epiphyses may be a feature of the disorder.[14]

Spherocytic anemia. Spherocytic anemia, also designated hereditary spherocytosis,

Fig. 10-4. A, Roentgenograms of the lower limb bones of another child with clinical thalassemia. Also evident here are thinning of the cortices of the tibia and fibula, some distension or flaring of the metaphyseal portions of the tibia, and distinct alteration of the architecture of the cancellous bone. The changes are present in all the bones but are more pronounced in the long limb bones and in the metatarsals (not shown). **B,** The upper limb bones in the case illustrated in **A.** The changes already cited are again evident in all the bones but are particularly striking in the metacarpals and phalanges.

familial hemolytic anemia, and chronic hemolytic jaundice, is characterized by spherocytosis; increased fragility of the red cells to hemolytic agents, especially to hypotonic salt solution; moderate hemolytic anemia; icterus (slight to moderate, except after hemolytic crises); and splenomegaly, often quite marked.

As its various names indicate, the disorder is chronic, congenital, and often familial. There are records of many families in which jaundice has existed through several generations. While the condition is transmitted through male and female descendants alike, not all of the children in a family are affected. Although the disease has been known clinically for a long time, the precise nature of the erythrocytic defect or abnormality in biochemical terms has not yet been elucidated. The jaundice may be noted shortly after birth or later,

at any time during childhood, but it may be so slight as to escape recognition until adult life. Many affected persons live to an advanced age.

In keeping with the relative mildness of the disorder, as compared with the other chronic hemolytic anemias, skeletal changes of the nature previously described (Figs. 10-2 to 10-4) are absent or equivocal in most cases, although some instances have been recorded in which alterations in the skull and limb bones were as pronounced and extensive as in thalassemia. Also noteworthy are certain developmental anomalies that occur often enough to suggest that they are not fortuitous, but rather result from the gene defect. Oxycephaly (tower skull, turmschädel) in particular has often been noted, as have abnormalities in the eyes, the root of the nose, the palate, the teeth, and the fingers.

References

1. Wintrobe, M. M.: Clinical hematology, ed. 6, Philadelphia, 1967, Lea & Febiger.
2. Caffey, J.: Pediatric x-ray diagnosis, ed. 5, Chicago, 1967, Year Book Medical Publishers.
3. Lichtenstein, L.: Bone tumors, ed. 3, St. Louis, 1965, The C. V. Mosby Co.
4. Stern, C.: Principles of human genetics, San Francisco, 1949, W. H. Freeman & Co.
5. Brinkhous, K. M., editor: Hemophilia and other hemorrhagic states, Chapel Hill, 1959, University of North Carolina Press.
6. Seegers, W. H.: Blood coagulation in hemophilia B, Bull. Path., October, 1968, p. 199.
7. Thomas, H. B.: Some orthopaedic findings in 98 cases of hemophilia, J. Bone Joint Surg. **18**:140, 1936.
8. Ghormley, R. K., and Clegg, R. S.: Bone and joint changes in hemophilia with report of cases of so-called hemophilic pseudotumor, J. Bone Joint Surg. **30-A**:589, 1948.
9. Freund, E.: Die Gelenkerkrankung der Bluter, Virch. Arch. Path. Anat. **256**:158, 1925.
10. Brinkhous, K. M., Shanbrom, E., Roberts, H. R., Webster, W. P., Fekete, L., and Wagner, R. H.: A new high-potency glycine-precipitated antihemophilic factor (AHF) concentrate, J.A.M.A. **205**:615, 1968.
11. Schaaf, W. J.: Early aspiration of joint in Christmas disease, J.A.M.A. **175**:509, 1961.
12. Pauling, L., Itano, H. A., Singer, S. J., and Wells, T. C.: Sickle cell anemia, a molecular disease, Science **110**:543, 1949.
13. Gabuzda, T. G., Nathan, D. G., and Gardner, F. H.: Thalassemia trait: genetic combinations of increased fetal and A_2 hemoglobins, New Eng. J. Med. **270**:1212, 1964.
14. Currarino, G., and Erlandson, M. E.: Premature fusion of epiphyses in Cooley's anemia, Radiology **83**:656, 1964.

General reference

Moseley, J. E.: Bone changes in hematologic disorders (roentgen aspects), New York, 1968, Grune and Stratton, Inc.

Chapter 11

Paget's disease of bone (osteitis deformans)

Paget's disease of bone

Paget's disease is a not uncommon condition that has tantalizingly eluded full clarification, although we have learned a great deal about its manifestations over the years. We know from physiologic investigation that active lesions of Paget's disease show significant hypervascularity and, collaterally, from radioisotope tracer studies, that they manifest greatly accelerated metabolic turnover. This may have its reflection clinically in wide pulse pressure and peripheral signs of high cardiac output. We know, on the other hand, from the valuable investigation of Schmorl,[1] that subclinical lesions of limited extent, involving particularly portions of the sacrum and/or lumbar vertebrae, actually outnumber those in the pelvis, skull, long limb bones, and other sites, producing symptoms. (The incidence of Paget lesions, including the silent ones in the vertebral column, was over 3% in a sizable series of subjects past 40 years of age, whose skeletons were thoroughly examined at autopsy.)

We have learned to recognize most lesions of Paget's disease roentgenographically, although some of the early lesions and those in unusual locations may present a problem for the inexpert (Figs. 11-1 and 11-2). We are well aware that sarcoma

may develop in established clinical lesions of Paget's disease, with significant though not alarming frequency,[2] and that, curiously enough, benign giant cell tumors may make their appearance, especially in the calvarium and facial bones.[3,4]

We know that, pathologically, the initial expression of the disorder is a localized area of resorption (whether it be in the calvarium, tibia, humerus, or some other bone). This localized lesion is followed by repeated alternating cycles of bone formation and renewed resorption over a period of several or many years, leading eventually to readily recognizable gross alterations of architecture and, microscopically, to a unique complex structural pattern of bone designated "mosaic" by Schmorl.[1] However, when it comes to the basic question of what initiates or is responsible for this sequence of changes, we actually know little more than did Sir James Paget[5] in 1877 when he described a group of advanced cases in point as "osteitis deformans"; we have not advanced beyond the stage of speculation[6] (Fig. 11-3).

Clinical considerations. Paget's disease is observed mainly in middle-aged or older patients, although occasional instances may be encountered in individuals below the age of 40.[3,7] I have seen a remarkable set

122

Fig. 11-1. Roentgenogram showing an expanded lesion of Paget's disease in the sternal end of a clavicle.

Fig. 11-2. Roentgenogram showing early (monostotic) Paget involvement in a proximal ulna. A film taken 4 months earlier showed a transverse pathologic fracture (now healed). Biopsy showed a richly vascular lesion of Paget's disease in an early resorptive phase.

123

Fig. 11-3. Photographs of an elderly patient with widespread, advanced Paget's disease. Note the enlarged head, kyphosis with foreshortened barrel chest, bowing of the femora and tibiae, and marked widening and deformity of the tibiae, especially the left tibia.

of roentgenograms showing well-developed, unmistakable changes of Paget's disease in the long limb bones of both upper and lower extremities, pelvis, and lumbar spine of a young man, aged 18, who had complained of bone pain for some 3 years previously (Fig. 11-4). It may be noted, on the other hand, that most cases of so-called juvenile Paget's disease in the older literature apparently represent instances of fibrous dysplasia. Familial incidence has been observed but is exceptional.[8]

The only laboratory aid to diagnosis is estimation of serum alkaline phosphatase activity, which is consistently elevated in Paget's disease, even when it is localized. When Paget's disease is complicated by osteogenic sarcoma, one may get fantastically high levels, exceeding those in any other condition.

The condition may develop in one, several, or many bones. While symptomatic lesions predilect the calvarium, the innominate bones, the vertebral column, and the long limb bones, one may occasionally find them in such sites as the sternum, clavicle, and hand and foot bones. Although there is wide variation in the extent and tempo of the disease, the usual history is one of slow progress over a period of many years. By the same token, the condition is compatible with long life, so that most patients die of natural causes rather than from bone sarcoma, cardiovascular disease, or other sequelae of Paget's disease. However, it should be emphasized that not all cases of

Fig. 11-4. An extraordinary instance of Paget's disease, widespread and full-blown in a patient, age 18.

Paget's disease show steady progression to an advanced stage, and the spontaneous healing tendency in the condition is well known.[3,9]

Pain is often, though not necessarily, an early distressing symptom, especially in the low back (Fig. 11-5) or in a bone of a lower extremity, particularly the tibia. Symptomatic relief has been noted,[3] though not consistently, after the administration of a variety of remedies, including androgen (to men) and estrogen (to women) in the same doses that one would use for osteoporosis. These hormones also tend to reverse hypercalcuria, when present. For refractory pain not responding to any other measures, small fractional doses of x-ray irradiation may be effective, perhaps because it tends to reduce vascularity. Large dosage, however, is contraindicated and may induce a pathologic fracture that will not heal.

Other manifestations that may require orthopedic or medical attention are bowing of the femur or tibia, infractions (particularly transverse fissure fractures on the convex side of bowed bones), urolithiasis (from hypercalcuria), and sometimes deafness, blindness, or proptosis from pronounced thickening of the skull. Because of the hazard of hypercalcuria and stone formation, one should avoid immobilization, high calcium diet, and vitamin D. If immobilization is required temporarily, calcium should be limited and fluid intake kept high, to avoid potentially serious hypercalcemia.

Both multiple myeloma and hyperparathyroidism have been noted to occur in association with Paget's disease of bone, but this appears to be coincidental or fortuitous.

Pathologic changes. As indicated, sizable circumscribed rarefied skeletal defects reflect the early resorptive changes in Paget's disease. Their appearance and significance in the calvarium (Fig. 11-6) are well recognized (so-called osteoporosis circumscripta cranii).[10] Comparable defects may, of course, develop in other bones—an innominate bone, a tibia, or a humerus—as a forerunner of typical Paget transformation. When a tibia is involved, it is fre-

quently the upper half of the shaft that is altered, although occasionally the lower end may display comparable changes (Fig. 11-7). While the rarefied defect often appears to terminate sharply, the process tends to progress along the shaft and is likely to be associated with some expansion of the bone and thinning of its cortex. Although there is not, as yet, any discernible coarse trabecular architecture, even at this stage of evolution, the microscopic changes observed in a biopsy specimen can be readily identified as those of Paget's disease (Fig. 11-8).

Whatever the site of early or initial resorption, it is apparently brought about by inordinate vascularity and, even more so, by intense osteoclastic activity (far exceeding that seen in hyperparathyroidism, for example). The resorbed bone is inevitably replaced by fibrous tissue, in which

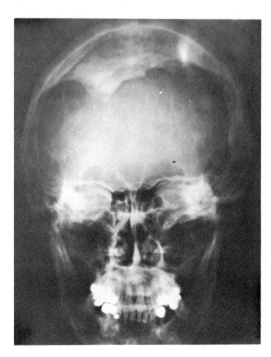

Fig. 11-5. Roentgenogram showing Paget alteration in a single, somewhat flattened and broadened vertebral body. (There was persistent pain but not nerve root compression.)

Fig. 11-6. Roentgenogram of a skull showing huge lucent areas of rarefaction reflecting the early resorptive phase of Paget's disease (so-called osteoporosis circumscripta cranii).

Fig. 11-7. **A,** Roentgenogram of a lesion of early Paget's disease in a lower tibia, which is still in a resorptive stage. Note the advancing cortical resorption at the proximal limit of the lesion. **B,** Roentgenogram of another lesion of relatively early (monostotic) Paget's disease in a distal tibia, showing a pathologic fracture through its proximal end.

Fig. 11-8. Photomicrograph of an early Paget lesion showing extensive resorption of the cortical bone, replacement by vascular connective tissue, intense osteoclastic activity, and numerous small trabeculae of new bone rimmed by osteoblasts.

Fig. 11-9. Photomicrograph of a representative field from a biopsy of a tibial cortex showing a later stage of Paget's disease. In the bone at the lower left one sees the development of a mosaic pattern (numerous small irregular bits of bone, outlined by conspicuous cement lines). This pattern can be accentuated by polarized light. On the cortical surface (top), there are layers of reconstructed new bone.

new bone is laid down by proliferating osteoblasts (Fig. 11-8). This, in turn, undergoes resorption. Thus the cycle goes on and on, until eventually the bone presents a peculiar complex pattern described by Schmorl as "mosaic." It no longer has an orderly lamellar structure but instead is composed of irregular bits and pieces of bone, demarcated by unusually prominent cement lines (Fig. 11-9). It should be emphasized, however, that this jigsaw or mosaic architecture is a feature of advanced or late Paget transformation and, as such, is

not a sine qua non for diagnosis in biopsy specimens, for example.

Grossly, transformed Paget bone presents a peculiar coarsened trabecular architecture, which is brought out particularly well in macerated preparations and, of course, is reflected roentgenographically (Fig. 11-10). The new bone is deposited endosteally and to some extent within the general medullary cavity and is also irregularly laid down by the periosteum, so that the surface of the affected bone appears rough and pumice-like. In the process there is an

Fig. 11-10. Roentgenogram of a late or advanced lesion of Paget's disease in a tibia showing marked widening of the shaft and typical coarse trabecular architectural alteration. The latter is also evident in the calcaneus. Compare with Fig. 11-7, which shows an earlier stage in the evolution of the condition.

Fig. 11-11. Roentgenogram of a portion of the shaft of a tibia (obtained as an autopsy specimen) showing pronounced thickening and other changes of late Paget's disease.

Fig. 11-12. **A,** Roentgenogram of a strikingly thickened and enlarged skull in a later stage of Paget's disease (so-called cotton-wool calvarium) showing transformation of its tables and relatively dense areas of new bone formation irregularly interspersed among more lucent areas of resorption. **B,** Frontal section through a calvarium showing pronounced thickening from Paget's disease in its posterior half (top of figure). The anterior half was uninvolved and serves as a normal control for comparison.

appreciable increase in the width of the bone (Fig. 11-11). Further, since this porous bone lacks customary structural strength and solidity, it is not only vulnerable to infraction but also yields under stress, so that the development of such deformities as tibial and femoral bowing, coxa vara, and kyphoscoliosis (sometimes with cord compression) is quite understandable. In the skull, pronounced calvarial thickening as a late or end stage (Fig. 11-12) may lead to special problems (apart from headache) resulting from encroachment on the auditory canal, cochlea, or orbit. Also, in some instances a cosmetic problem is created by concomitant involvement of facial bones and maxillae (but not the mandible, as a rule).

For a meticulously detailed account of the pathologic anatomy of Paget bone, the natural tendency to healing, and the unusual development of osteosclerosis as an end stage, the reader may have profitable recourse to the articles of Jaffe[9,11] dating back to 1933. For highlights of some of the relevant clinical problems, as well as pathologic features, the richly illustrated paper of Goldenberg[3] is recommended.

Malignant change in Paget's disease. The problem of sarcoma developing in Paget's disease is an important one and has received considerable attention in recent years.[2] Sarcoma is usually observed in patients with fairly extensive Paget's disease of long standing, but it may occur even in monostotic Paget's disease. Commonly, it is some one bone that manifests malignant change. This is shown roentgenographically by the appearance of an ominous rarefied defect that had not been previously noted. However, it is not at all unusual to observe the development of two or more sarcomas simultaneously within bones transformed by Paget's disease, such as in the calvarium and in one or more of the large limb bones, particularly the femur, tibia, and humerus (Fig. 11-13).

The neoplasm that develops is most often an osteogenic sarcoma, but it need not be that. It may prove to be fibrosarcoma or an anaplastic tumor containing many multinuclear tumor cells, so as to simulate malignant giant cell tumor. The development of chondrosarcoma in Paget bone has also been observed,[3] although this is distinctly unusual. Whatever the type of

Fig. 11-13. A broadened and deformed femur of an old man with extensive Paget's disease who developed bone sarcoma in both lower extremities.

131

sarcoma, it grows rapidly and metastasizes early, as a rule, so that the prognosis is distinctly bad. There are relatively few survivors beyond 1 year or less, even after well-conceived, prompt radical surgery.

Other hyperostoses affecting the skull particularly

There are many diverse conditions that may lead to localized thickening of the calvarium, facial bones, and/or jaw bones.

Hyperostosis frontalis interna, as its name clearly indicates, is characterized by irregular thickening of the inner table of the frontal bone and is sometimes observed in older women, possibly reflecting endocrine (estrogen) imbalance.

Osteomata may occasionally present on the outer surface of the calvarium as circumscribed, rounded, ivory-like exostoses, but more often they are found protruding into the orbit or one of the paranasal sinuses. If one examines such an osteoma before it is fully evolved, it is seen to be composed of prominent plaques and trabeculae of new bone within a benign osteoblastic connective tissue matrix.[2]

Localized gigantism, which may on rare occasions affect the skull and contiguous soft parts, is an example of a developmental anomaly producing asymmetrical enlargement and distortion.

Tumors, especially meningiomas, may also be responsible for localized hyperostosis of the calvarium. An appreciable number of meningiomas penetrate the dura and invade the overlying bone, and occasionally the reactive osteosclerosis that ensues may be sufficiently pronounced to produce a prominent, tumor-like protuberance ("meningeom-hyperostose").[12] On the other hand, meningioma en plaque extensively invading the calvarium may sometimes have a striking lytic effect on the bone. I have seen a case in point in which, over a period of several years, virtually the entire anterior half of the calvarium disappeared radiographically. A focus of myeloma in the calvarium may sometimes produce not the customary rarefied defect but rather reactive osteosclerosis with perpendicular orientation of the new bone striae to the tables, so that the roentgenogram simulates that of reaction to a meningioma.

Fibrous dysplasia is still another condition that may bring about a sizable, localized, blister-like expansion of the outer table of the calvarium, although more often it induces thickening of the bones at the base of the skull. It may manifest itself in deforming localized expansion of one or both of the jaw bones, especially in young patients.

Symmetrical enlargement of the mandibles and distinctive eye changes may be observed in the peculiar localized developmental disorder known as *cherubism.*

Congenital syphilis may sometimes result in pronounced skeletal hyperostoses. In these circumstances, parts of the skull and facial bones (as well as the limb bones) may become abnormally thick and dense. This unusual picture is said to be similar to that in certain cases of *goundou.*[13]

In some instances of *Paget's disease,* the skull, facial bones, and maxillae alone are affected. (Such cases were at one time thought to represent leontiasis ossea.)

There may well be additional unusual causes of hyperostosis and transformation of one or another part of the skull, but the long list that has been presented will suffice to indicate that the problem in differential diagnosis can be quite complex.

Instances of slowly developing, more generalized thickening of the facial bones, often associated with comparable changes in the lower jaw and cranium (not resulting from any of the specific conditions previously mentioned) have for a long time been designated as *leontiasis ossea.*[14,15] The swelling and deformity of these bones, depending on their extent, may or may not result in nasal obstruction, proptosis, or impairment of vision. Leontiasis ossea, however, is not a pathologic entity. It appears rather to represent a miscellaneous category, of which some components are not as well understood as they might be. Some instances in point apparently result from a spreading, sclerosing, inflammatory osteoperiostitis (thought possibly to be infectious, but actually of obscure nature). Others are associated with polyposis of the colon and soft tissue tumors and have a familial pattern,[16] apparently indicative of a peculiar developmental disorder predicated on a gene defect. In still others, the thickened bones are said to be rarefied rather than sclerotic, and there is apparently no significant inflammatory reaction ("infection") in evidence. What the latter cases represent, no one knows.

That familial hyperostosis of the skull and facial bones can occur without associated intestinal polyposis or other apparent anomalies is evidenced by a case in point seen by me in consultation in 1955 for Dr. E. C. H. Lehmann of Vancouver, British Columbia.[17] In this family, three siblings presented unusual, diffuse thickening of the facial bones and of the skull, especially along its base (Fig. 11-14). Biopsy of the parietal bone of one of the children, then 6 years of age, showed great thickening of the bone without any significant alteration in its histologic pattern. Comparable involvement (seen roentgenographically) of the calvarium, facial bones, and mandible, as well as of other extracranial bones (ribs, clavicles, metacarpals, metatarsals, phalanges, and so forth) has been reported by van Buchem and his associates[18] under the title of "Hyperostosis Corticalis Generalisata." It is noteworthy that of their seven patients there was a set of twins and another pair of siblings. More recently, Fosmoe, Holm, and Hildreth[19] reported the roentgenographic findings in another case (in an adult) of even greater extent and severity under the heading of van Buchem's disease. Whether the cases presenting familial cranial hyperostosis exclusively and those presenting extracranial skeletal involvement as well are closely related would appear to be a moot point at this time.

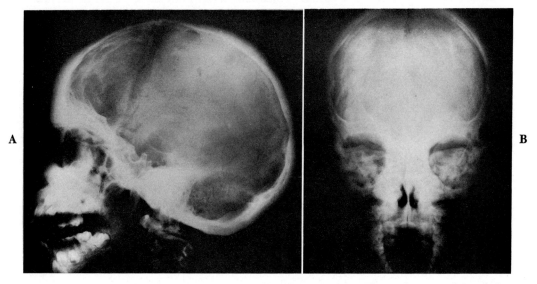

Fig. 11-14. Lateral and anteroposterior views showing the striking changes of familial hyperostosis of the skull and facial bones. Two other children in the family showed similar changes. (Courtesy Dr. E. C. H. Lehmann, Vancouver, British Columbia.)

References

1. Schmorl, G.: Über osteitis deformans Paget, Virch. Arch. Path. Anat. **283**:694, 1932.
2. Lichtenstein, L.: Bone tumors, ed. 3, St. Louis, 1965, The C. V. Mosby Co.
3. Goldenberg, R. R.: The skeleton in Paget's disease, Bull. Hosp. Joint Dis. **12**:229, 1951.
4. Hutter, R. V. P., Foote, F. W., Jr., Frazell, E. L., and Francis, K. C.: Giant cell tumors complicating Paget's disease of bone, Cancer **16**:1044, 1963.
5. Paget, J.: Trans. Roy. Chir. Soc. London **60**:37, 1877.
6. Reifenstein, E. C., Jr., and Albright, F.: Paget's disease: a concept as to its pathologic physiology and the importance of this in the complication arising from fracture and immobilization, New Eng. J. Med. **231**:525, 1944.
7. Wagner, M.: Report of case of Paget's disease in 18-year-old male, with review of literature, Wisconsin Med. J. **46**:1098, 1947.
8. Evens, R. G., and Bartter, F. C.: The hereditary aspects of Paget's disease (osteitis deformans), J.A.M.A. **205**:900, 1968.
9. Jaffe, H. L.: Paget's disease of bone, Arch. Path. **15**:83, 1933. (Contains a survey of pathologic alterations.)
10. Erdheim, J.: Über die genese der Paget schen Knochenerkrankeng, Beitr. Path. Anat. Path. **96**:1, 1935.
11. Jaffe, H. L.: Atypical form of Paget's disease appearing as generalized osteosclerosis, Arch. Path. **16**:769, 1933.
12. Oehlecker, F.: Eine ungewöhnliche Geschwülst des Schädeldaches (Meningeom-Hyperostose), Zbl. Chir. **34**:1433, 1952.
13. Hodges, P. C., Phemister, D. B., and Brunschwig, A.: The roentgen-ray diagnosis of diseases of the bones and joints, New York, 1938, Thomas Nelson & Sons, p. 44.
14. Evans, J.: Leontiasis ossea: a critical review with report of 4 original cases, J. Bone Joint Surg. **35-B**:229, 1953.
15. Fairbanks, H. A. T.: An atlas of general affections of the skeleton, Edinburgh, 1951, E. & S. Livingstone Ltd., pp. 206-208.
16. Plenk, H. P., and Gardner, E. J.: Osteomatosis (leontiasis ossea): hereditary disease of membranous bone formation associated in one family with polyposis of the colon, Radiology **62**:830, 1954.
17. Lehmann, E. C. H.: Familial hyperostosis of the skull and facial bones, J. Bone Joint Surg. **39-B**:313, 1957.
18. Van Buchem, F. S., Hadders, H. N., Hansen, J. F., and Woldring, M. G.: Hyperostosis corticalis generalisata: report of seven cases, Amer. J. Med. **33**:387, 1962.
19. Fosmoe, R. J., Holm, R. S., and Hildreth, R. C.: Van Buchem's disease (hyperostosis corticalis generalisata familiaris), Radiology **90**:771, 1968.

Chapter 12

Histiocytosis X

(eosinophilic granuloma, Letterer-Siwe disease, and Schüller-Christian disease)

The integrated concept[1-5] of eosinophilic granuloma of bone, Letterer-Siwe disease, and Schüller-Christian disease as interrelated manifestations of a single nosologic entity has gained wide acceptance in recent years. The name "histiocytosis X," proposed by me[2] in 1953 as a provisional broad general designation for this malady, likewise appears to be taking hold. For an account of the historic development of this concept to which many American and European investigators have contributed, for the detailed pathologic evidence in its support, and for convenient clinical orientation including discussion of specific indications for rational therapy, the reader may have recourse to critical reviews on the subject published in 1953 and 1964, respectively.[2,5]

The interrelationship of the various clinical and pathologic manifestations is outlined in the following classification of histiocytosis X, first set forth[2] in 1953. The recognized types of clinical involvement can be grouped under the general heading and still be differentiated from one another, so that useful distinctions having a bearing on treatment and prognosis are maintained.

Classification of histiocytosis X

I. Histiocytosis X, localized to bone (eosinophilic granuloma, solitary or multiple)

II. Histiocytosis X, disseminated, acute or subacute (Letterer-Siwe syndrome)
  With destructive skeletal lesions (eosinophilic granuloma)
  With transition to chronic phase (Schüller-Christian disease)

III. Histiocytosis X, disseminated, chronic (Schüller-Christian syndrome)
  With destructive skeletal lesions (eosinophilic granuloma)
  With early extraskeletal lesions (indicate sites) resembling eosinophilic granuloma
  With acute or subacute exacerbation (Letterer-Siwe disease)
  With involvement predominantly of bones, lungs, pituitary, and/or brain, skin, mucous membranes (oral, anal, genital), liver or lymph nodes, and so on (in varying combinations, as the case may be)

There can no longer be any doubt that Letterer-Siwe disease and Schüller-Christian disease represent acute (or subacute) and chronic expressions, respectively, of the disseminated form of the malady. In this connection, it must be recognized that both these eponyms were adopted as convenient provisional designations for ostensibly finite clinical syndromes at a time when their intimate relationship could hardly be suspected. In other ways also, our concept of the conditions so designated has broadened in scope far beyond any-

135

Fig. 12-1. Photomicrograph of a liver biopsy from an adult with long-standing chronic disseminated histiocytosis in recrudescence (he had had recurring osseous, buccal, and cutaneous lesions over a period of some 15 years). Note the small bile duct (at the top) surrounded by an involuting histiocytic nodule (containing some eosinophils) and enveloped by inflammatory scar tissue. In its vicinity, one also sees proliferating bile ducts and markedly distended bile canaliculi (going on in the other areas to bile lakes). (×90.)

thing the authors concerned could ever envision.

As for the lesion of eosinophilic granuloma, it seems clear from pathologic evidence now available that it represents the pathologic expression of early, rapidly developing reaction to the etiologic agent, whatever it may ultimately prove to be. As such, it may appear not only within bone, where its presence was first recognized,[6] but also in many other sites, notably in lymph nodes, oral cavity (gingiva, palate, and so on), and anogenital region, as well as in the lungs, thymus, liver, kidneys, female genitalia, and possibly the eye and cranial nerves (in time, there will undoubtedly be other additions). Further, the lesion of eosinophilic granuloma may also appear in the lungs, liver, bones, and other sites as the pathologic expression of recrudescence in well-established, chronic, disseminated histiocytosis X, even of long standing (Fig. 12-1).

In regard to the etiology of histiocytosis X, I still favor infection, conceivably of viral nature, as a more plausible explanation than any alternative. Although no specific infectious agent has been identified, there are indirect clinical indications suggesting infection, notably the bouts of fever associated at times with the appearance of fresh lesions in bone and other sites; the fever, night sweats, and loss of weight associated with the onset of severe pulmonary involvement in some cases, so that the initial clinical impression is active tuberculosis; and the spread of lesions in skin and bone to regional lymph nodes.[5] Further, I have seen material from a case of eosinophilic granuloma in the skull of a teen-age girl whose father also developed a focus of eosinophilic granuloma in the skull the following year. These are admittedly only straws in the wind, but they all seem to lean in the same direction. The question of an infectious origin should undoubtedly be investigated with modern techniques of virus culture, tissue culture, and electron microscopy.

The discussion that follows represents essentially a digest of the views expressed in previous articles on the subject by myself and my colleagues,[1-5] especially the reviews published in 1953[2] and 1964.[5] My observations since then have served to confirm the usefulness of these concepts as a basis for comprehensive orientation. I have not found it necessary to postulate atypical or transition forms of the disorder to explain the clinical and pathologic findings in any given case, as was the vogue some years ago. The extensive literature has further substantiated these views and broadened their scope.

Eosinophilic granuloma of bone (histiocytosis X localized in bone)

The mildest and most favorable expression of the disease (histiocytosis X) is represented by cases presenting one, several, or occasionally many destructive foci within the skeleton, and otherwise showing neither apparent constitutional indications of illness nor any discernible evidence of cutaneous, pulmonary, hypophyseal, or other extraskeletal involvement. The pathologically descriptive name "eosinophilic granuloma of bone"[6] still seems to be an appropriate designation for such instances, which merit special consideration by virtue

Fig. 12-2. Roentgenogram of a solitary focus of eosinophilic granuloma in the lower shaft of the humerus of a child, 2 years of age, who had restricted motion and some tenderness for about 2 months. The lesion was thought to be a tumor and the affected segment of the bone was resected (good reconstruction was obtained by the use of a tibial graft reinforced by abundant cancellous bone from the iliac crest). Had the diagnosis been established at the time of surgery by frozen section, thorough curettement and packing would have sufficed for cure.

of their auspicious prognosis. I am inclined to regard this skeletal localization as an indication of successful confinement of the etiologic agent, which may well account for the favorable outcome. One can venture a good prognosis for recovery in such cases, even though an appreciable number of skeletal lesions are present and even

Fig. 12-3. Roentgenogram of a lesion of eosinophilic granuloma in the intertrochanteric region of a femur in a child, which was thought to be a bone cyst before surgery. Cure was obtained by thorough curettement and packing with bone chips. (No additional foci were found on skeletal survey.)

though additional skeletal lesions subsequently make their appearance, as occasionally happens.

In the matter of clinical diagnosis, it is worth emphasizing again that a focus of eosinophilic granuloma of bone is prone to develop so rapidly and to break through the cortex of the affected bone so readily that, prior to biopsy, it is often mistaken clinically for a primary malignant tumor, especially Ewing's sarcoma (Fig. 12-2). By the same token, comparable multiple foci appearing in the skeleton of a child, for example, may conceivably give rise to the initial impression of metastatic neuroblastoma. Despite their seemingly ominous behavior, however, it is well known that such lesions heal readily following curettement or roentgen therapy (in relatively small dosage). It has also been demonstrated[1] that they may even regress or disappear spontaneously.

It is also important to emphasize that, in actual practice, it is not always possible on initial examination, especially in a young child, to be certain that skeletal lesions pathologically identified as eosinophilic granuloma do not have their histiocytic counterpart elsewhere, or that extraskeletal lesions will not manifest themselves subsequently, even though at the time roentgenographic examination of the chest

Fig. 12-4. Roentgenogram of a calvarial defect that proved to be a focus of eosinophilic granuloma. This is a common site of localization. (To venture any opinion as to prognosis, one would have to know whether the disease was disseminated or confined to bone.)

Fig. 12-5. Roentgenogram of a rarefied lesion of eosinophilic granuloma in the body of the tenth thoracic vertebra of an adult, who also presented additional foci in several other bones as well as difuse bilateral pulmonary infiltration indicative of chronic disseminated histiocytosis X. (The importance of a chest film and of thorough physical examination in such patients must be emphasized.) The skeletal lesions were effectively controlled by roentgen therapy in comparatively small dosage.

is negative and physical examination fails to reveal involvement of the skin, mucous membranes, or hemopoietic organs. To be more explicit, inasmuch as the pathologic lesion of eosinophilic granuloma of bone represents the expression of acute skeletal involvement in the disease as a whole (histiocytosis X), whether this be localized or disseminated, it follows that from the roentgenogram of such a lesion, or even from a biopsy of it alone, one cannot make any reliable forecast as to prognosis, since this depends largely upon whether there is associated visceral involvement and more particularly upon the distribution, extent, and severity of these visceral lesions. In certain instances, it may be necessary to re-

serve judgment and to follow the patient closely for a number of months or even for several years. In particular, the clinician must be on the alert for such indications as fatigability, chronic malnutrition, loss of weight, slight fever, predisposition to secondary infections, and the frequent appearance of new skeletal defects as harbingers of systemic involvement of potentially serious import.

Today experienced radiologists are very likely to consider the possibility of eosinophilic granuloma in the differential diagnosis of rapidly developing, destructive le-

Fig. 12-6. Photomicrograph of a well-preserved field in a lesion of eosinophilic granuloma of bone. The leukocytes massed on the left are all eosinophils, many of them young forms. The large pale cells to the right are of histiocytic nature. (×450.)

sions of bone (Figs. 12-2 to 12-5). Recognition of the lesion by pathologists in most instances occasions little difficulty, even when the histologic picture is altered by extensive hemorrhage and necrosis with giant cell reaction. When the diagnosis is missed or is not clear at the onset, it is generally for one of two reasons. First, prolonged acid treatment of the surgical specimen for decalcification interferes with the staining of the eosinophilic granules within leukocytes—whenever possible, bits of soft tissue not requiring decalcification should be processed separately. Second, lesions that are operated relatively late may be extensively modified by pathologic fracture, cortical perforation, scarring, and periosteal new bone reaction. In these circumstances, one may have to scrutinize all available tissue fragments closely for telltale foci of eosinophilic granuloma featuring proliferating histiocytes admixed with clumps of eosinophils (Figs. 12-6 and 12-7, *A*).

With reference to age incidence, eosinophilic granuloma of bone may occasionally affect infants as well as older children and adults. In older adults, a lesion of eosinophilic granuloma (in a rib, for example) may be asymptomatic. The most common sites of localization are the limb bones, skull, vertebral column, and innominate bone (Figs. 12-2 to 12-5), but the lesion may be encountered elsewhere.

When eosinophilic granuloma localizes in a vertebral body, it may lead to compression fracture with pronounced flattening and, sometimes, to spinal cord or nerve root impingement. In children, this may develop insidiously without early detection. Vertebra plana (Calvé's disease), long thought to result from avascular ne-

Fig. 12-7. **A,** Section of an eosinophilic granuloma in the frontal bone of a 15-year-old boy. (×470.) **B,** From an enlarged cervical lymph node in the case illustrated in **A** showing the picture of eosinophilic granuloma on the left and residual lymphoid tissue on the right, for contrast.

crosis, is commonly a sequel of eosinophilic granuloma.

Acute (or subacute) disseminated histiocytosis X (Letterer-Siwe syndrome)

Before instituting treatment or venturing an opinion as to prognosis, one should be certain of the diagnosis on pathologic as well as clinical grounds. It must be borne in mind that the German pediatrician Siwe described only a clinical syndrome rather than a pathologic entity. It so happens that the same combination of clinical manifestations may be caused not only by acute dis-

Fig. 12-8. Photomicrograph of a lymph node also involved by eosinophilic granuloma (from another case). Note the focal nodular aggregates of histiocytes; the small dark cells within these nodules are eosinophils. (Low magnification.)

seminated histiocytosis X but also by neoplastic reticulosis (or reticuloendotheliosis) with or without associated leukemia. Obviously, one must resort to biopsy whenever possible to distinguish the two. Thus a young child with a destructive focus of eosinophilic granuloma in bone (Fig. 12-6), mucocutaneous lesions showing histiocytic proliferation (with or without associated eosinophil reaction), enlarged lymph nodes showing focal nodular histiocytosis (Fig. 12-8), and bone marrow that fails to show any neoplastic growth can, with assurance, be said to be suffering from acute (or subacute) disseminated histiocytosis X, rather than from something akin to acute leukemia. Adequate steroid therapy for such a child may well be lifesaving if the disease is not fulminant, whereas the use of marrow-damaging cytotoxic agents,

like nitrogen mustard, or of radioactive elements might well have serious consequences.

Acute or subacute disseminated histiocytosis X may be observed occasionally in adults as well as young children. The condition, although serious, is not necessarily fatal, as was once thought. With improved therapy, an appreciable number of patients have remissions of significant duration and presumably go into the chronic phase of the disease (Schüller-Christian). Attention has been directed particularly to the use of selected antibiotics to control secondary bacterial infections and to the value of steroid therapy in critical situations. Autopsy experience indicates that when the outcome is fatal despite well-conceived therapy, it is usually because the disease is fulminant or because of unresponsive secondary infection, extensive pulmonary in-

Fig. 12-9. Roentgenogram showing old dense infiltration of both lung fields in a young man of 29, who had also had symptoms of diabetes insipidus for about 4 years and then developed a lesion of eosinophilic granuloma in the calvarium. (From Lichtenstein, L.: Histiocytosis X, Arch. Path. **56:**84, 1953.)

volvement, or serious hepatic damage leading to cirrhosis.

Chronic disseminated histiocytosis X (Schüller-Christian disease)

The following concepts concerning the chronic form of histiocytosis X may be re-emphasized[5] here in outline form for the sake of brevity.

1. The old belief that chronic histiocytosis X represents a primary disorder of lipid metabolism (or a functional disturbance of the reticuloendothelial system) should be discarded as no longer having any justification.

2. Only a small minority of patients, perhaps no more than one in ten, manifests the complete Christian triad—calvarial defects, exophthalmos, and diabetes insipidus.

3. Skeletal lesions should no longer be considered to be a sine qua non for the diagnosis, since they may be absent or, if they do appear, they may not become manifest until lesions in extraskeletal sites (such as the lungs) are already well established (Fig. 12-9).

4. Although the clinical picture may vary considerably from case to case, all manifestations fit within a unified framework of reference as clinical expressions of chronic disseminated histiocytosis X, of which the tempo, severity, and localization may vary within wide limits. The major types of involvement are skeletal, pulmonary, cutaneous, and hypophyseal (or cerebral).

When the condition proves fatal, as it may in adults, as well as children, it is usu-

Fig. 12-10. Photomicrograph of an old sclerotized lesion in the tibia of an adult who presented no clinical manifestations of extraskeletal involvement (burned out or healed end stage of Schüller-Christian disease). Note the presence of numerous lipophages and collagen-forming fibroblasts in the tissue between the sclerotic trabeculae of spongy bone. This is the picture once referred to as "lipoid granulomatosis." (From Lichtenstein, L.: Histiocytosis X, Arch. Path. **56**:84, 1953.)

ally for one of the following reasons: acute or florid exacerbation, extensive pituitary damage (in cases manifesting diabetes insipidus), progressive pulmonary disease leading to honeycomb lungs and resulting cor pulmonale, or hepatic involvement resulting in intrahepatic obstructive jaundice and eventually cirrhosis (if the patient survives long enough).

5. The intial pathologic picture is essentially that of an inflammatory histiocytosis that may or may not be accompanied by intense eosinophil reaction. Fibrosis and conversion of histiocytes to lipophages are secondary, if not late, changes (Fig. 12-10).

6. Finally—and this of prime importance —early, rapidly developing lesions as seen in biopsy specimens commonly have the characteristics of eosinophilic granuloma.

This is true not only in bone but also in skin, oral cavity (gingiva, palate, or tongue), anogenital region, lungs, lymph nodes, liver, kidney, and other sites.

Of particular interest are the observations showing that the early disseminated nodular lesions in the lungs resemble eosinophilic granuloma. This is apparently an important portal of entry of the etiologic agent (Fig. 12-11). Similarly, the early lesions in the liver around portal radicles likewise have the character of eosinophilic granuloma and may lead rather rapidly to serious intrahepatic obstructive jaundice[4] (Fig. 12-1). Also noteworthy are the observations[5] indicating that lesions of eosinophilic granuloma in bone, as well as in the cutis, may extend to regional lymph nodes (Fig. 12-7, *B*).

Fig. 12-11. Photomicrograph of a pulmonary lesion of eosinophilic granuloma, showing replacement of pulmonary parenchyma by histiocytes interspersed with eosinophilic leukocytes. (The smaller dark cells are young eosinophils, many of them uninuclear or bilobed.)

In the matter of treatment, one may stress the established value of roentgen irradiation (in limited dosage) in the control of osseous and mucocutaneous lesions, particularly, adequate therapy for the control of diabetes insipidus (when present), and the usefulness of steroids for pulmonary involvement, especially in its early stage and for critical exacerbation in general.

References

1. Jaffe, H. L., and Lichtenstein, L.: Eosinophilic granuloma of bone: a condition affecting one, several or many bones, but apparently limited to the skeleton, and representing the mildest clinical expression of the peculiar inflammatory histiocytosis also underlying Letterer-Siwe disease and Schüller-Christian disease, Arch. Path. **37**:99, 1944.

2. Lichtenstein, L.: Histiocytosis X: integration of eosinophilic granuloma of bone, "Letterer-Siwe disease" and "Schüller-Christian disease" as related manifestations of a single nosologic entity, Arch. Path. **56**:84, 1953.

3. Lichtenstein, L.: Medical progress, pathology: diseases of bone, New Eng. J. Med. **255**:427, 1956.

4. Parker, J. W., and Lichtenstein, L.: Severe hepatic involvement in chronic disseminated histiocytosis X, Amer. J. Clin. Path. **40**:624, 1963.

5. Lichtenstein, L.: Histiocytosis X (eosinophilic granuloma of bone, Letterer-Siwe disease, and Schüller-Christian disease): further observations of pathological and clinical importance, J. Bone Joint Surg. **46-A**:76, 1964.

6. Lichtenstein, L., and Jaffe, H. L.: Eosinophilic granuloma of bone, Amer. J. Path. **16**:595, 1940.

Chapter 13

Chemical and radiation effects on bone

Chemical effects on bone

With reference to chemical damage, apart from benzol poisoning (which can cause aplastic anemia), we are concerned here mainly with the pathologic effects of certain chemical elements, some of which have been well documented in the past as important industrial hazards. This concise survey will deal only with the manifestations in bone. For discussion of the other noxious systemic effects of these chemical agents, the reader may have recourse to standard reference texts on toxicology and internal medicine.

In chronic *lead* poisoning (plumbism, saturnism), the heavy metal is stored in bone or in other depots (brain, kidneys, and liver). In limb bones specifically, it tends to be concentrated in the ends of the bone. In affected adults (painters, pottery workers, white-lead workers, and others), this deposition does not cause any apparent untoward effects except for anemia and a bluish line along the gums adjacent to the teeth. In children (who ingest lead-containing paint on their cribs or even the walls), one characteristically sees a transverse radiopaque line or band on the metaphyseal side of the growth plates of the long limb bones (Fig. 13-1). The width of this dense zone radiographically indicates

the duration of exposure to lead. Its appearance apparently reflects abnormally condensed, calcified cartilage and newly formed bone, rather than the presence of lead itself.[1]

After the administration of *bismuth* to babies (or experimental young animals[2]), one also sees transverse dense bands in the juxtaepiphyseal regions of long bones, although this observation is only of historic interest now that penicillin has replaced bismuth in the treatment of congenital syphilis. As in the case of comparable lead lines, the radiopaque zones contain abundant compacted calcified cartilage, reflecting interference with orderly endochondral ossification. As these zones later move away from the growth plate and undergo reconstruction, they remain relatively dense for some time.

Still another chemical agent that may produce radiopaque bands in or adjacent to the growth zones of long bones in babies or children is *phosphorus*, which was once used (as yellow phosphorus or phosphorized cod liver oil) in the treatment of rickets.[3] As an industrial poison, yellow phosphorus (in workers in match factories, particularly) was once responsible for more or less extensive necrosis of the jaw bones and refractory osteomyelitis, sometimes leading

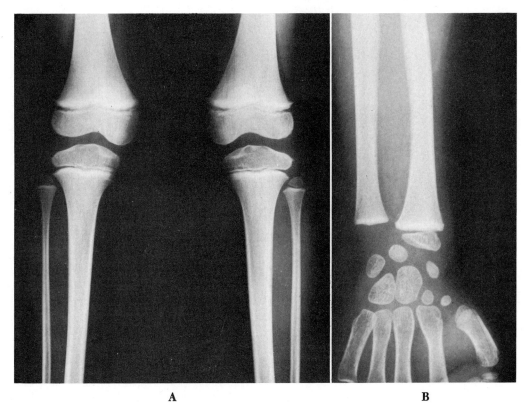

A   **B**

Fig. 13-1. **A,** Roentgenogram showing transverse lead lines at the growth plates of a child (who had ingested lead paint on its crib). **B,** Comparable changes in the distal radius and ulna.

to massive sequestration and involucrum.

It now appears to be established from statistical surveys that the addition of *fluoride* to drinking water in minute concentration reduces the incidence of dental caries. It is currently claimed in television commercials that its addition to toothpaste accomplishes the same end ("Look, Daddy, only one cavity"). Be that as it may, excessive intake of fluorine has deleterious skeletal effects. Excessive fluoride content in water in certain endemic areas where fluorosis is prevalent, such as parts of Texas and Oklahoma, may lead to mottling of the tooth enamel in growing children. In comparable adults, and also in rock miners who have ingested large amounts of fluoride as an occupational hazard (cryolite and certain phosphate rock miners), more or less striking, diffuse osteosclerosis develops from both endosteal and periosteal apposition.[4,5] The earliest changes of fluoride osteosclerosis are said to occur in the lumbar spine and pelvis.[5] There is often calcification of the neighboring tendons and ligaments, including the pelvic and vertebral longitudinal ligaments, associated with osteosclerosis. On microscopic examination of the bone, all one sees is abnormally dense bone, without anything distinctive otherwise (Fig. 13-2).

Mercury poisoning is far less common than it was when mercurial drugs and ointments were used in the treatment of syphilis. It is still seen as an industrial disease or, very occasionally, following attempts at suicide with mercuric bichloride. (Today, people jump off the Golden Gate

147

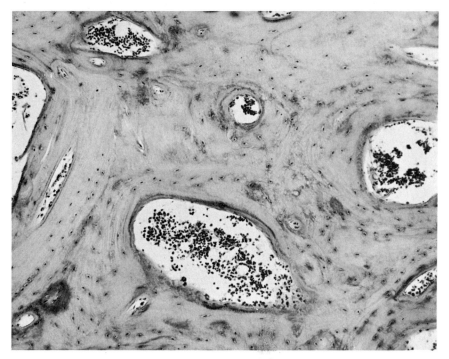

Fig. 13-2. Photomicrograph showing abnormally dense bone (osteosclerosis), as seen in fluoride poisoning.

Bridge instead.) The only skeletal effect, if it can be called that, is loosening of the teeth.

It may be mentioned here that *beryllium*, when implanted in bone experimentally or administered intravenously,[6] provokes reactive osteosclerosis leading to the development of osteogenic sarcoma. This observation is of greater academic interest than practical moment.

Radiation effects on bone

Occasional exposure to small doses of *roentgen rays* (delivered by well-calibrated and supervised equipment) in the course of diagnostic procedures is not held to be harmful. Repeated exposure over a long period of time, even when the usual safeguards are observed, may be a hazard—radiologists are more prone to develop leukemia than are other physicians. The possibility of the insidious induction of gene mu-

tations in these circumstances has also been raised by concerned biologists and geneticists, although this still appears to be a moot point.

Roentgen irradiation in heavy doses employed in therapy[7] (for the destruction or control of neoplasms particularly) regularly induces certain well-recognized pathologic changes in tissues within the beam of irradiation, including bone. The major effects are the following: calcification (Fig. 13-3), narrowing or obliteration of blood vessels, necrosis or necrobiosis, scarring and hyalinization, and, in the reparative phase, the appearance of abnormal fibroblasts with large swollen nuclei. Still larger or massive doses may, of course, be followed by obvious gross changes as well, including destruction and ulceration of the skin, necrosis of soft tissues (including muscle) in the irradiated field, and partial necrosis in the bone itself.

Fig 13-3. Photomicrograph of a representative field of a lesion of Paget's disease in a tibia, which had been heavily irradiated on the mistaken premise that it represented a malignant tumor (pathologic fracture and nonunion developed and the leg was eventually amputated). The intense calcification of Paget bone and the necrobiosis in places are postirradiation changes.

Another important consideration is the occasional development of sarcoma in bone or soft tissues following therapeutic irradiation[8] after a latent interval that may be as short as 3 years or as long as 20 to 30 years or more. When postirradiation sarcoma develops in bone, it is most often an osteogenic sarcoma, but it may be fibrosarcoma or even chondrosarcoma. As a rule, the hazard is directly proportional to the dosage employed, athough there are undoubtedly exceptions. With increasing recognition of such cases, there has been a growing feeling, first, that nonneoplastic lesions in bone or in joints should be treated by irradiation only when there is a clear, specific indication for it, and second, that when irradiation is preferred, whatever the reason may be (and this applies also to tumors), one

should use the smallest dose calculated to be effective.

Certain radioactive elements, including radium, mesothorium, plutonium, and strontium[90], may cause the development of bone sarcoma. Osteogenic sarcoma has been induced experimentally, for example, by the administration of radium[9] (in rats), by exposure to plutonium (also in rats), and to radiostrontium (in mice). As for tumor induction in man, Evans and his associates,[10] following up the pioneer study of radium (and mesothorium) watch-dial painters by Martland,[11] observed a 10% incidence (as of 1964) of osteogenic sarcoma in persons who had had symptomatic radium poisoning. Other significant long-term sequelae were focal necrosis and eventual loss of teeth, radiographically mottled areas

149

of radiation necrosis and "osteitis" that are prone to fracture, osteomyelitis (of the jaw bones, particularly), and, in a few instances, carcinoma of the paranasal sinuses or mastoid.

These investigators pointed out, further, that radium and mesothorium are deposited in bone in an irregular pattern, with "hot" spots in metabolically active areas that contain a hundred times the concentration of radioactivity found in adjacent areas of bone. Inasmuch as these deposits, small as they may be, set up a never-ending alpha particle bombardment over a long period of time, one may have justifiable concern about the long-term effects of radioactive fallout, especially that of the bone-seeking radioactive elements, such as plutonium or strontium[90]. It is quite conceivable that we may yet witness a significant rise in the incidence of osteogenic sarcoma, as well as of leukemia, and that we may have to revise our present estimates of what constitutes a "safe" concentration of radioactive fallout. The next 10 years should tell the story.

References

1. Caffey, J.: Clinical and experimental lead poisoning: some roentgenologic and anatomic changes in growing bones, Radiology 17:957, 1931.
2. Caffey, J.: Changes in growing skeleton after administration of bismuth, Amer. J. Dis. Child. 53:56, 1937.
3. Phemister, D. B., Miller, E. M., and Bonar, P. E.: Effects of phosphorus in rickets, J.A.M.A. 70:850, 1921.
4. Møller, P. F., and Gudjonsson, S. V.: Massive fluorosis of bones and ligaments, Acta Radiol. 13:269, 1932.
5. Stevenson, C. A., and Watson, A. R.: Fluoride osteosclerosis, Amer. J. Roentgen. 78:13, 1957.
6. Kelly, P. J., Janes, J. M., and Peterson, L. F. A.: The effect of beryllium on bone, J. Bone Joint Surg. 43-A:829, 1961.
7. Rubin, P., and Casarett, G. W.: Clinical radiation pathology, Philadelphia, 1968, W. B. Saunders Co.
8. Hatcher, C. H.: Development of sarcoma in bone subjected to roentgen or radium irradiation, J. Bone Joint Surg. 27:179, 1945.
9. Dunlap, C. E., Aub, J. C., Evans, R. D., and Harris, R. S.: Transplantable osteogenic sarcomas induced in rats by feeding radium, Amer. J. Path. 20:1, 1944.
10. Gary, G. E., Clark, S. D., and Evans, R. D.: Radium and mesothorium poisoning in human beings: report of over 375 cases, presented at American Medical Association meeting, San Francisco, June, 1964.
11. Martland, H. S.: Occurrence of malignancy in radioactive persons: a general review of data gathered in the study of the radium dial painters, with special reference to the occurrence of osteogenic sarcoma and the inter-relationship of certain blood diseases, Amer. J. Cancer 15:2435, 1931.

Chapter 14

Pathology of some common and unusual orthopedic conditions

This section will deal with some thirty miscellaneous, more or less common orthopedic conditions not considered in preceding chapters. It is concerned mainly with "bread and butter" orthopedic pathology and puts together for convenient reference observations that, though generally well known, may not be readily available elsewhere.

Pathology of menisci of the knee

Lacerated meniscus. The crescent-shaped menisci serve presumably as shock absorbers. Though commonly referred to as "cartilages," they are actually composed of dense collagenous connective tissue. As sports buffs are well aware, they are often torn following injury to the knee and must then be removed before damage to other articular structures ensues. Because of their limited blood supply, spontaneous repair or healing of menisci following laceration is apt to be so slight as to be negligible. Extensive injury may lead to complete bucket-handle tear (Fig. 14-1, *A*), but less extensive types of laceration are also commonly observed (Fig. 14-1, *B* and *C*). When a meniscus "regenerates" following removal, it takes the form usually of a fibrous cord. Calcification of meniscal connective tissue is seen only infrequently.

Sections for microscopic examination are best taken in a vertical plane at right angles to the site of apparent or suspected laceration. As a rule, they show nothing more striking than degeneration and fraying or fibrillization of the connective tissue and, sometimes, slight focal capillary vascularization as well. Needless to say, it is essential for the examining pathologist to distinguish clearly the irregularly roughened, modified tract of an injury from the clear, sharp, inadvertent cut of the surgeon's scalpel.

Discoid meniscus. Discoid meniscus manifesting an anomalous broadened structure (as its name implies) is of practical moment in that it is peculiarly vulnerable to horizontal splitting (Fig. 14-2).

Meniscal or parameniscal cysts. Meniscal cysts result from focal myxoid degeneration and cystic softening of meniscal collagenous connective tissue, usually toward the meniscocapsular junction. In many ways, their formation is reminiscent of the way in which a ganglion develops: there is a tendency for the multifocal cystic areas to coalesce (Fig. 14-3), and occasionally a sizable, clinically evident mass may be formed. I have seen a specimen of a cyst of a lateral meniscus of a knee, containing colorless viscid fluid, that had attained the size of a fist.

151

Fig. 14-2. Photograph of a surgically removed, discoid meniscus of a knee.

Fig. 14-1. A, Photograph of a lacerated meniscus of a knee, showing a bucket-handle tear. B and C, Other examples of torn menisci.

Fig. 14-3. A, Photograph of a cyst of a medial meniscus (external view). B, Section of the specimen illustrated in A.

Chronic bursitis

Chronically irritated bursal sacs develop with great frequency in many paraskeletal sites, particularly where there has been friction between apposing gliding surfaces or over bony prominences (housemaid's knee and philosopher's elbow, for example, have become colloquialisms). Such sacs are commonly operated because of swelling and/or painful motion. At such sites, the connective tissue undergoes appreciable thickening and encompasses a cyst-like space containing mucinous fluid.

The lining of the sac may come to resemble synovium, but this is not necessarily so. In any event, the lining usually presents irregular ridges and small nodular excres-cences, often discolored yellow-brown by hemosiderin pigment. There may also be deposits of fibrinoid material on or within the lining surface; its organization often leads to fibrous strands or cords traversing the lumen of the bursal sac (Fig. 14-4, A). It is not uncommon also to find fibrin rice bodies attached to the lining or lying free within the sac. Very occasionally, calcified

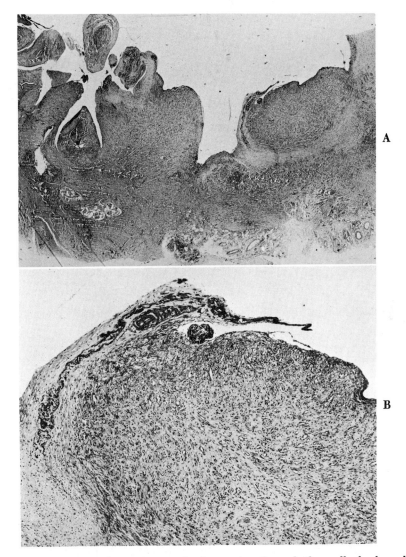

Fig. 14-4. A, Low power photomicrograph of a section through the wall of a bursal sac. B, Higher magnification of an area of the lining of the bursal sac illustrated in A, showing intense capillary vascularization as well as organizing fibrin on its surface.

chondral bodies resembling joint mice are encountered.

These features are, of course, evident in microscopic sections, which, in addition, show more or less intense vascularization of the lining by innumerable sprouting capillaries (Fig. 14-4, B). Despite the common designation of bursitis, there is usually no inflammatory exudative reaction.

Ganglion formation

The common ganglion develops through myxoid degeneration and cystic softening of the collagenous connective tissue of a joint capsule or tendon sheath. As such, it constitutes a "tumor" only in the limited clinical sense of a swelling (Fig. 14-5, A). As in comparable multilocular cyst formation within parameniscal connective tissue of the knee joint, it enlarges and ramifies through coalescence of areas of cystic change (Fig. 14-5, *B*). Obviously, crushing of a ganglion alone will not prevent its reappearance, since it does not remove the connective tissue implicated in its formation.

Herniated intervertebral disk tissue

Surgery for ostensibly herniated intervertebral disk tissue impinging on nerve roots has become a major stock in trade for neurosurgeons and some orthopedists, although there are many who feel that it is undertaken too often. Be that as it may, the sur-

Fig. 14-5. **A,** Low power photomicrograph showing ganglion formation through myxoid change and cystic softening of the collagenous connective tissue of a joint capsule (in the wrist region). (×8.) **B,** Photomicrograph of another ganglion showing its multilocular structure. The spaces contained colorless, viscid fluid in the gross. (×9.)

Fig. 14-6. A, Photomicrograph of a bit of (herniated) intervertebral disk tissue removed surgically. The resemblance of the nuclei to those of cartilage cells is only superficial. (Actually, the cells of the nucleus pulposus are of notochordal derivation.) **B,** Photomicrograph showing protrusion of disk tissue, through a hiatus, into a vertebral body and its walling-off by a thin plate of bone (Schmorl's node).

gical pathologist, even in a smaller general hospital, has ample opportunity to learn to identify bits of intervertebral disk tissue and to distinguish these from cartilage, anulus fibrosus, ligamentum flavum, and so forth.

In examining intervertebral disk tissue fragments microscopically, one is not justified in stating that they are necessarily herniated, since the validity of this observation depends essentially on what is seen directly at the operating table. Nor is one justified ordinarily in stating that the intervertebral disk tissue submitted shows evidence of injury (unless there has been reparative vascularization) or that it shows significant degenerative change (since this inference would require elaborate controls with reference to age, occupation, body build, previous history, and so on that are not readily available). In most instances, all one can say in effect with any assurance is that Kilroy was there (Fig. 14-6, *A*).

As Schmorl, the distinguished German bone pathologist, demonstrated many years ago, herniation of intervertebral disk tissue into adjacent vertebral bodies is often seen on examination of the vertebral column at autopsy,. although it is asymptomatic and apparently of no practical consequence. Fig. 14-6, *B* shows a so-called Schmorl's node that has become walled-off by a thin plate of bone, as is usually the case.

One occasionally observes herniation of the intervertebral disk ventrally or anteriorly. This, too, is apparently asymptomatic, although it tends to provoke reactive new bone formation leading to a conspicuous radiopaque beak-like protrusion, which may appear curious and puzzling to those unfamiliar with it.

Pathologic changes in tendons and their sheaths

Many of the conditions that affect synovial joints have their counterpart in tendon sheaths (as well as bursae mucosae); the pathologic reaction is similar, whatever the localization. Thus one may encounter tenosynovial tuberculosis, chronic nonspecific

Fig. 14-7. Calcium deposition in a supraspinatous tendon.

inflammation (at the wrists, for example), rheumatoid inflammation, and, on occasion, even sarcoid. With reference to the last, I have observed a remarkable instance of sarcoid that involved primarily the tendon sheaths, rather than the usual sites (skin, lymph nodes, and bone, among others). Continuing the analogy, chondromatosis of tendon sheaths also occurs, as does commonly pigmented nodular tenosynovitis (formerly designated "giant cell tumor" of the tendon sheath). These lesions will be considered further on in relation to the pathology of synovial joints. (See Chapter 15.)

There are several noteworthy conditions affecting the collagenous connective tissue of tendons. Chief among them is *calcification*. This is seen most often in the supraspinatous tendon (and frequently in the subdeltoid bursa, as well), but on occasion it may also involve other tendons, such as the patellar, gluteus, peroneus, and flexor carpi ulnaris. The pathogenesis of this calcium deposition is still moot, although there

has been much speculation about it. Examination of surgical specimens from cases in point may show some degeneration of collagenous connective tissue or even focal necrobiosis, but I have not seen significant necrosis that might conceivably account for calcification as a sequel (Fig. 14-7).

In the shoulder region particularly, calcification is often painful and may require aspiration, cortisone injection, x-ray therapy, or other modalities for relief. As a rule, it is self-limited, but occasionally the problem may become a persistent one. In general, it may be observed that the paraskeletal collagenous connective tissue structures (and this applies to joint capsules and ligaments as well as tendons) have a meager blood supply and thus usually require 3, 4, or even 6 months for an injury to heal and for concomitant relief of symptoms, regardless of what is done by way of treatment.

Localized calcification in soft parts—of the fingers, for example—may occur quite apart from calcification in tendons. Interest-

A   B

Fig. 14-8. Roentgenograms showing calcinosis of fingers in association with scleroderma.

Fig. 14-9. A, Photomicrograph showing degeneration of connective tissue in a tendon. **B,** Myxoid degeneration and cystic softening of tendinous connective tissue, as a forerunner of spontaneous rupture.

ingly enough, such calcinosis may occur in association with scleroderma (Fig. 14-8), but it may be encountered occasionally as an idiopathic manifestation. In the Burnett or milk-alkali syndrome[1] (seen in peptic ulcer patients), calcium deposits may also be laid down in skeletal structures, subcutaneous tissues, and the eye (band keratopathy); however, this is reversible.

Traumatic rupture of tendons is well

known, especially in football players who may sever their heel cords or plantaris or patellar tendons, for example. Tendons, particularly the Achilles tendon, may also undergo significant *degenerative change* (Fig. 14-9, *A*). When the process develops relatively slowly over a period of years and allows for irregular scarring, a swelling or pseudotumor may be the result. More often, there is peculiar myxoid degeneration and

Fig. 14-10. Photomicrograph of a section taken through a bulbous amputation neuroma.

cystic softening, for no apparent reason, predisposing to spontaneous rupture (Fig. 14-9, *B*).

Another condition that is noteworthy is *stenosing tenovaginitis*, particularly of a tendon sheath of a finger (so-called trigger finger). In this condition there is a block to the free movement of the tendon caused by a focal, nodular, fibrocartilagenous thickening of the tendon sheath, which must be excised to correct the condition.

Amputation neuroma

Amputation neuroma is a common cause of painful amputation stump, although it is also seen after the severance of peripheral nerves that are not repaired promptly and effectively for whatever reason. When explored, an amputation neuroma presents as a focal bulbous swelling at the site of severance. On microscopic examination one sees smaller and larger proliferating nerve bundles enveloped in scar tissue; these pre-

sumably fail to join their counterparts (Fig. 14-10).

Volkmann's contracture

Volkmann's contracture is the common orthopedic designation for contracture of muscle tissue following a deep laceration in which nutrient blood vessels are severed —for example, in the forearm, after the hand is thrust through a plateglass window. What happens pathologically is that, as a sequel of muscle necrosis, tracts of fibrous tissue grow into the muscle by way of attempted repair (Fig. 14-11). Whatever deformity ensues is the result of contraction of this scar tissue.

Dupuytren's contracture

Dupuytren's contracture is a fairly common surgical condition resulting from fibroplasia (or fibromatosis) of the palmar fascia—one of many sites of fibroplasia that may be encountered throughout the body.

159

Fig. 14-11. Photomicrograph illustrating the changes found in Volkmann's contracture. Note the tract of scar tissue within the field of necrotic muscle.

When the examining pathologist sections one or more of the gristly nodules in a relevant surgical specimen, he finds active spindle cell proliferation (Fig. 14-12), which may at times cause some concern over the possibility of fibrosarcoma.

Actually, the process is self-limited; I have seen hundreds of cases in point and have no knowledge of a single instance of malignant change. What happens is that these cellular foci subside and collagen is formed, which contributes to the thickening of the palmar fascia. Foci of active fibroplasia may, however, appear subsequently in other sites, accounting for the chronicity of the condition. This should not be con-

strued as recurrence in pathologic terms. The collagen deposited tends to contract, and when this occurs in the fascial slips that extend into the flexor surface of the fingers, the latter are drawn into the palm of the hand, producing the characteristic deformity that Dupuytren described.

Essentially the same process is encountered at times in the plantar fascia of one or both feet.[2,3] Focal nodular fibroplasia in this site, however, seldom leads to contracture, as it does in the hand. Complete excision of the plantar fascia may be required for the relief of tender or painful nodes and to prevent "recurrence."

It may be noted that fibroplasia or fibro-

Fig. 14-12. Photomicrograph showing a focus of active fibroplasia (in the palmar fascia of a patient with Dupuytren's contracture).

matosis may develop in the connective tissue of muscle as well as in fascia, such as in the abdominal wall ("desmoid"), thigh, and sternocleiodomastoid muscle of both newborn and older children. If the condition does not regress spontaneously in the last site listed, contracture of scar tissue may lead to the development of wryneck (*congenital torticollis, fibromatosis colli*).

Baker's cyst

The term "Baker's cyst" has come to be applied rather loosely to any cyst-like structure in the popliteal space. Sometimes the cyst results from a herniation of the posterior capsule of the knee joint, although communication with the joint cannot always be demonstrated. In these circumstances, the sac may have a thin wall, mucinous contents, and a delicate lining resembling synovium. Fibrous-walled bursal sacs in the popliteal area are also designated by some as Baker's cyst, although I do not follow this practice, preferring to avoid the

eponym altogether as being unnecessarily confusing.

Slipped capital femoral epiphysis

Slipped capital femoral epiphysis (adolescent coxa vara, coxa anteverta) is occasionally encountered as a spontaneous painful development in adolescents who tend to be overweight. Its pathogenesis has been the subject of much speculation for 30 years or more (Fig. 14-13). Adequate pathologic specimens are not readily available, inasmuch as the condition, if discovered early, may be corrected by closed manipulation. However, in the cases in which open surgery was done relatively early and sufficient bone was removed for pathologic examination, we had the distinct impression that the essential lesion was a shearing of the epiphyseal cartilage plate,[4] without necrosis, degeneration, or any other predisposing change, except perhaps for increased vascularity at the plate associated with a spurt of active growth at this period, as

161

Fig. 14-13. Roentgenogram showing slipped capital femoral epiphysis.

Fig. 14-14. Roentgenogram showing the changes of bilateral congenital coxa vara.

Trueta has emphasized. It is true that La-croix and Verbrugge,[5] from their examina-tion of a large specimen, postulated a fi-brous transformation at the plate as the basic change. However, the condition in their case had been present for 3 years be-fore a reconstructive procedure was done, and the changes they described may well have been secondary in nature.

Congenital coxa vara

Congenital coxa vara is another condition in which the capital femoral epiphyses are displaced, in varus position, presum-ably on the basis of a congenital ab-normality (Fig. 14-14). I have not had occasion to examine any specimens ob-tained during open corrective procedures and I am therefore not in a position to

Fig. 14-15. Roentgenograms showing the changes of Blount's disease.

comment on the essential pathology of the condition at first hand.

Blount's disease

Another condition that is well-known clinically but about which little is known pathologically is *Blount's disease,* which is characterized by maldevelopment and deformity of one side of the upper tibial epiphysis and contiguous metaphysis (Fig. 14-15).

Congenital pseudoarthrosis of tibia

Because it may be noted at birth or during childhood, pseudoarthrosis is held to be congenital. It is characterized clinically by thinning of the tibial cortex, predisposing to fracture through the shaft, and by a tendency to persistent fibrous union and pseudarthrosis, which is difficult to overcome surgically (Fig. 14-16). From the literature, it would appear that in about half of the cases reported there were cutaneous and other manifestations of von Recklinghausen's disease. In the specimens of connective tissue and bone obtained in the course of corrective surgical procedures that we have had

Fig. 14-16. Roentgenogram showing congenital pseudoarthrosis of the tibia in a child.

163

Fig. 14-17. Roentgenogram showing avascular necrosis of both femoral heads in caisson disease.

an opportunity to examine, we made it a point to search for indications of neurofibromatosis as a possible explanation for failure of bony union, but with no success.

Infarcts in bone

Inasmuch as the long limb bones are supplied by nutrient arteries with limited collateral circulation, it is not surprising that infarcts, particularly at the bone ends, are found in a variety of predisposing circumstances, although they are not nearly as common as infarcts in certain viscera (heart, spleen, and kidneys, for example).

Perhaps the most common cause of necrosis is loss of adequate blood supply following certain fractures, such as in the femoral head after fracture of the neck.

Fig. 14-18. An old infarct in the lower shaft of a femur—an incidental finding in an adult presenting an eosinophilic granuloma of a rib. There was a comparable symmetrical infarct in the opposite femur and similar smaller ones in both upper tibiae.

164

Apart from this, bone infarcts, notably in one or both femoral heads, are seen in caisson workers (sandhogs) and occasionally in high altitude military flyers, presumably as a result of air (gas) embolism (Fig. 14-17). They are observed also in Negroes with sickle cell anemia, apparently as a sequel of vascular occlusion. In patients with collagen disease, particularly disseminated lupus erythematosus, who have been on massive steroid therapy, infarcts of the femoral head have been noted too frequently for this to be fortuitous although pathologic evidence (of endarteritis) is hard to come by.

Embolism in cardiac patients (Fig. 14-19), especially those with rheumatic heart disease and auricular fibrillation, is still another cause of infarcts in bone. As previously noted (Chapter 6), deposition of abnormal lipid in the bone, especially of the femora in Gaucher's disease, may predispose to necrosis and particularly to collapse of the femoral head. Occasionally, infarction in the upper femur may be observed after injudicious forceful manipulation. From time to time, one may also observe old infarcts in bone that were clinically silent and for which there is no apparent cause (Fig. 14-18).

Whatever the cause of an infarct in bone, the involved area is, as a rule, readily recognizable in the gross as a well-demarcated, yellowish zone. In the femoral head, this often takes the form of a subchondral triangular wedge of varying size. A recent in-

Fig. 14-19. Photograph showing an old infarct of bone found at autopsy in the upper femur of a 70-year-old man with heart block. Microscopically there was extensive secondary cholesterol deposition within the area of necrosis.

Fig. 14-20. Roentgenogram showing linear calcification within the upper shaft of a humerus, which may reflect either an old infarct or a calcified enchondroma.

165

Fig. 14-21. Photomicrograph of an area of infarction (in a femoral head) showing necrosis of the bone and of the marrow as well. There was no creeping replacement or substitution of the dead bone in this field.

Fig. 14-22. Photomicrograph of an older area of infarction in which there has been appreciable calcification (black zones in the print) and organization of the necrotic marrow.

farct (in the femoral head, for example) stands out radiographically as a relatively radiopaque area (Fig. 14-17). This may reflect the fact that the area of avascular necrosis retains its original density, whereas the surrounding bone undergoes resorption, making for appreciable contrast. An older infarct (in a femoral shaft, for example) may have variable density; it stands out because of the irregular calcification within it (Figs. 14-18 and 14-22). It should be pointed out, however, that intramedullary calcification may also outline a calcified enchondroma. At times, the differentiation may be difficult without tissue examination (Fig. 14-20).

Microscopically, there are two cardinal features that characterize an infarct in bone:

1. Necrosis of the bone, as evidenced by the finding of empty lacunae devoid of osteocytes. This finding in itself is not sufficient, since it may follow a fracture.
2. The presence of necrotic detritus within the marrow spaces (Fig. 14-21).

An infarct in time tends to undergo certain secondary changes, namely scarring of the marrow, irregular calcification of dead bone and marrow, cholesterol deposition, and sometimes cystic softening (Fig. 14-22). With reference to the last, I have seen a specimen in point of a femoral head and neck in which there were cystic spaces up to 2 cm. in diameter containing clear viscid fluid. Reconstruction of the dead bone takes place, as previously noted (Chapter 1), by creeping replacement or substitution. Thin strips or tiers of new bone are deposited on top of the necrotic bone by osteoblasts accompanying vascular connective tissue that is able to penetrate the area of infarction. While this process is fairly rapid in a child (with Perthes' disease, for example), it is likely to be painfully slow in an adult; many years may be required for any meaningful reconstruction of an infarct.

Avascular necrosis of bone in "juvenile osteochondritis"

Infarcts of bone in so-called juvenile osteochondritis (epiphyseal osteochondritis of growth centers, osteochondritis deformans juvenilis, osteochondrosis, and so on) comprise a special category about which reams have been written, much of it speculative. The nomenclature is obviously misleading in that inflammation is not a feature of the process. To make the subject more confusing, a dozen or more eponyms have been employed over the years to denote essentially the same lesion in various locations. This

Fig. 14-23. Roentgenogram showing a small focus of osteochondritis dissecans in the medial femoral condyle of a child.

167

much is clear from pathologic evidence: irrespective of whatever primary or secondary epiphysis is affected, or whether a small circumscribed area or an entire epiphysis is involved, the essential change is one of avascular necrosis or infarction. Thus if one examines sections of an "osteochondritis dissecans" body from a knee joint, for example (Fig. 14-23)—and these are readily available as surgical specimens (either semidetached or as free joint bodies)—one finds necrosis of the subchondral bone and of the marrow as well (Fig. 14-24, *A*). The same is true of bone samples of the capital femoral epiphysis in Legg-Perthes' disease (Fig. 14-24, *B*). The cause of the infarct is pre

sumed to be interference with or loss of essential blood supply. This is a logical inference, although it is seldom, if ever, demonstrated pathologically. What is peculiar and puzzling is the phenomenon itself—why should infarcts develop in the growing epiphyses of young patients? Why, for example, should a circumscribed area of avascular necrosis appear in the capital femoral epiphysis (as shown in Fig. 14-25, *A*) or in both femoral heads (as illustrated in Fig. 14-25, *B*)? The answer apparently lies in the realm of pathophysiology of the available vasculature. Trueta has made many provocative relevant observations, which I shall not go into here.

A   B

Fig. 14-24. A, Photomicrograph of a representative field of an osteochondritis dissecans body, which was removed from a knee joint. The articular cartilage (above the dense horizontal cement line near the top) is viable. The subchondral bone, however, is substantially dead, and the marrow spaces within it contain dark-staining necrotic detritus. **B,** Roentgenogram of a child with Legg-Perthes' disease. Pathologic examination of the affected capital femoral epiphysis at this stage would demonstrate avascular necrosis, analogous to that shown in **A.**

Fig. 14-25. A, Roentgenogram of a circumscribed focus of osteochondritis dissecans on the articular surface of a femoral head. B, Comparable lesions of osteochondritis dissecans in both femoral heads. It is noteworthy that at least two other members of this family had the same condition.

Fig. 14-26. Photomicrograph of a representative section of a specimen removed in a case of Osgood-Schlatter's disease. Note that the tibial apophysis (lower left) does *not* show avascular necrosis. The essential change is rather that of injury and reparative vasculation of the connective tissue between the apophysis and the tibia proper (upper right).

Incidentally, *Osgood-Schlatter's disease* does *not* belong in this category, despite what may be read in the literature. Pathologic examination of intact surgical specimens fails to show avascular necrosis of the tibial apophysis. What one does find is evidence of injury and reparative vascularization, either at the insertion of the patellar tendon or in the connective tissue interface between the apophysis and the tibia proper (Fig. 14-26). Uhry[6] demonstrated this in 1944. His observations were later confirmed and amplified by La Zerte and Rapp.[7] However, it appears that once a mistaken im-

pression gets into the literature, it takes many years to eradicate it.

Posttraumatic rarefaction of bone

Following an acute trauma without fracture (and the injury need not be severe), one occasionally sees not only atrophic soft tissue changes including muscle atrophy but also pronounced local rarefaction of bone. The "acute atrophy of bone" in these circumstances is accompanied by refractory pain and disability, which may persist for many months or even several years. Such changes in the hand and foot bones particu-

170

larly are commonly designated as *Sudeck's atrophy.*[8] They are reflected roentgenographically in a hazy appearance initially and later by a mottled or spotted rarefaction. The type and extent of the atrophy and the attendant disability go far beyond anything that might be ascribed to the simple atrophy of inactivity or disuse. Occasionally, the rarefaction may be more circumscribed and affect a scaphoid, semilunar, or ulnar styloid.

Comparable changes may appear after an injury in vertebral bodies, which are then prone to collapse insidiously, giving rise to so-called *Kümmell's disease.* Once in a while, posttraumatic rarefaction may develop in a large limb bone, especially the femur, and the roentgenographic changes may be sufficiently pronounced as to suggest infection or a bone tumor. It has been shown pathologically by Jaffe[9] and others that the mottled bone rarefaction seen radiologically reflects thinning and porosity of the compact cortical bone, as well as diminution in the size and number of the spongy trabeculae, and that these changes are associated with striking hypervascularity. The latter is particularly prominent in the cortical bone, where large resorption spaces around eroded haversian systems are filled with loose connective tissue in which numerous dilated and engorged blood vessels are present. As for pathogenesis of the condition, it is generally postulated, in keeping with the view of Leriche, that after a trauma there is initially a vasomotor reflex spasm with injury to one or more bones, followed by a loss of neurovascular tone, persistent vasodilation, and rapid vascular resorption of bone as a consequence.

It is conceivable that so-called *disappearing* or *vanishing bone disease* (phantom bones, massive osteolysis, regional angiomatosis) represents a more severe expression of the same phenomenon, rather than angiomatosis in the sense of a neoplasm, as some have suggested. This peculiar condition has been known clinically for a long time,[10] but it was not until recent years that a spate of articles on the subject appeared, only a few of which are cited here for convenient orientation.[11-14] Disappearing bone disease may affect one or more bones of the shoulder girdle (clavicle, scapula, and upper humerus), the lower extremity, and the pelvis, as well as ribs and vertebrae. Whatever region is involved, there is a tendency to progressive rarefaction and, eventually, lysis of the bone, so that its original contour is no longer discernible. Interestingly enough, the process tends to subside after a time, according to published reports, but not until there has been considerable loss of bone.

In the limited relevant material that I have had occasion to review, the only consistent feature was the presence of congeries of congested capillaries. While one can readily understand how this finding might be construed as indicative of hemangioma or "angiomatosis," I see no compelling reason to do so. There is a vast capillary bed in the marrow, only a small part of which is utilized or even discernible under ordinary circumstances. However, with loss of the normal neurovascular regulatory mechanism, the dilatation and engorgement of the entire potential capillary bed might easily simulate hemangioma.

Spondylolisthesis

Spondylolisthesis (slipping vertebra) or displacement of the vertebral column—commonly occurring at the lumbosacral joint, less often at L4-L5, and only occasionally at more proximal levels—is associated with a defect between the inferior and superior articular surfaces of the neural arch.[15,16] When there is separation of the neural arch without slipping, the condition is designated as *spondylolysis.* As Colonna[15] has indicated, the condition may go unrecognized in many patients without slipping or with only mild displacement, although the mechanical instability eventually predisposes to the changes of painful osteoarthritis.

171

These isthmic defects are believed by many to be of congenital origin, but Collonna favors the view that the condition is initiated by trauma at birth and aggravated by trauma in adult life. In any event, it appears that many patients are benefited by well-conceived nonsurgical measures. Spine fusion is reserved for stabilization of cases with prolonged severe low back pain that does not respond to conservative treatment.

Myositis ossificans

Myositis ossificans is actually a misnomer in that (1) inflammatory reaction is the ex-

Fig. 14-27. Roentgenogram showing an organized focus of myositis ossificans in the vicinity of an elbow joint, a relatively frequent site of localization.

Fig. 14-28. Photomicrograph of a lesion of myositis ossificans still in an active stage. Pictures such as this are sometimes interpreted as osteogenic sarcoma by inexperienced pathologists, who fail to take cognizance of the fact that the process has developed *outside* the bone.

ception, rather than the rule, and (2) it is the connective tissue in muscle that ossifies—the muscle tissue itself undergoes atrophy and tends to disappear at the affected site. In pathologic terms, the process is that of metaplastic ossification and sometimes cartilage formation as well in the connective tissue of muscle.

The condition is usually localized and is only rarely progressive or generalized. It occurs in children as well as adults. The most common sites of involvement are the thigh (in quadriceps and vastus muscles, particularly) and the arm (especially in the brachialis anticus muscle), although these are by no means the only ones (Fig. 14-27).

Very often there is a history of prior injury, but this is not invariably the case. Initially, there is a painful swelling of varying size, which can be puzzling or alarming clinically. Only after some 2 weeks or more does one discern focal radiopacity (reflecting bone formation through calcification of osteoid).

When the lesion is deep-seated and in proximity to the periosteum, its early roentgenographic picture may arouse a suspicion of malignant neoplasm, although it tends to become smaller and more clearly localized in the ensuing months. Malignant change in myositis ossificans has been recorded, but it is comparatively rare. As ex-

Fig. 14-29. Photomicrograph of an older, mature or reconstructed focus of metaplastic ossification of the connective tissue in muscle (myositis ossificans).

perienced orthopedists are well aware, early surgery before the process has become quiescent and static only tends to stir up renewed activity.

Examination of a surgical specimen of a focus of myositis ossificans still in an active phase reveals impressive proliferation of spindle connective tissue cells and, in places, the formation of osteoid and bone, which tends to become organized into trabeculae (Fig. 14-28). In this milieu, one can readily discern the transition from fibroblasts to osteoblasts. A small amount of cartilage may also be formed; this tends to undergo fairly rapid osseous transformation. In some lesions, giant cells may be prominent in places within the condensed connective tissue areas, as well as in proximity to mineralized matrix. The trabecular organization of bone is most apparent in the older peripheral portion of the lesion. This should be reassuring to a pathologist who is concerned about the possibility of osteogenic sarcoma, apart from the fact that the stroma, while cellular, is not malignant.

In older, mature, or reconstructed lesions of myositis ossificans in which the process has simmered down, active fibroplasia is no longer in evidence, and the bone that has been formed appears to be well organized (Fig. 14-29).

Metaplastic ossification in other sites

Viewed in perspective, myositis ossificans is only one expression of a more general phenomenon in skeletal pathology. Paraskeletal connective tissue, wherever it may be, retains the capacity to form bone and cartilage by metaplasia (perhaps this an atavistic throwback to the time when our remote ancestors were armadillos). This trait is apparently more pronounced in some individuals than in others. Thus one observes metaplastic bone, and perhaps cartilage, formation in joint capsules (either spontaneously or, more often, after surgery), in tendons (particularly the Achilles tendon, after injury or previous surgery),

in ligaments, fasciae, and aponeuroses, and, most importantly, in the cambium layer of the periosteum (after fracture and under other circumstances, to be indicated).

Periosteal ossification may follow an injury without fracture that results in a tear or lifting up of the membrane. It may also be a sequel of subperiosteal hemorrhage, notably in scurvy, hemophilia, or trauma ("ossifying hematomas"). Further, any intramedullary lesion of bone that erodes or penetrates the cortex stimulates the periosteum to lay down new bone in an apparent attempt to buttress the weakened bone. Oc-

Fig. 14-30. Roentgenogram showing a localized area of periosteal new bone apposition in the lower metaphysis of the femur of a teenager. There was some concern initially over the possibility of osteogenic sarcoma, but follow-up films taken 3 months later showed subsidence of the lesion and its gradual incorporation in the old cortex.

casionally, localized perioseal ossification develops without any obvious predisposing cause and may arouse concern over the possibility of osteogenic sarcoma (Fig. 14-30).

Subungual exostosis represents another noteworthy expression of metaplastic bone and cartilage formation by the cambium layer of the periosteum. In this condition, as the name indicates, a hard growth develops in the nail bed (of a toe), which protrudes from the dorsum of the distal phalanx (Fig. 14-31). Over the years I have had occasion to review a substantial number of instances submitted for opinion. In most of them, curiously enough, the patients were young females between the ages of 6 and 20 years— it may be that wearing open-toe shoes predisposes to injury at a time when the periosteum at this site is still potentially active. Be that as it may, sections show the "tumor" to be composed of actively growing, metaplastic bone and cartilage (in varying proportions), which is clearly of periosteal origin. When the process is exuberant, the examining pathologist, if he is not familiar with the condition, may take too serious a view of the findings and may interpret them as indicating osteosarcoma or chondrosarcoma. Actually, I have never seen malignant change in these circumstances.

In *hypertrophic osteoarthropathy,*[17,18] which is associated mainly but not exclusively with pulmonary neoplastic or suppurative disease, the periosteal new bone apposition is more widespread (Fig. 14-32) and may well reflect increased arterial pressure and blood flow, as Mendlowitz[19] has demonstrated.

Unicameral bone cyst

My interest in unicameral bone cyst, a not uncommon entity, dates back to 1942 when, in collaboration with Jaffe,[20] I described its essential pathology in correlation with the roentgenographic changes, with a view to resolving further the then popular mishmash of "localized fibrocystic disease of bone." It is noteworthy to see that with the delineation of fibrous dysplasia, bone cyst, and fibrous cortical defect or

Fig. 14-31. Roentgenogram of a well-established subungual exostosis protruding from the nail bed of the distal phalanx of a toe in a young patient.

Fig. 14-32. An instance of hypertrophic osteoarthropathy showing conspicuous periosteal new bone apposition on the lower tibia and fibula.

175

Fig. 14-33. Roentgenogram of a solitary unicameral bone cyst in its most common site, the upper metaphysis of a humerus. It still borders on the growth plate and is therefore in an active stage, capable of further enlargement.

Fig. 14-34. Roentgenogram of a unicameral bone cyst in the upper femur of a young woman of 22, which came to clinical notice because of a pathologic fracture of the femoral neck.

Fig. 14-35. A bone cyst in the lower shaft of the ulna in a child—a rather unusual site for it. This cyst was known to have been present for several years before it was operated.

nonossifying fibroma, as well as the osseous manifestations of hyperparathyroidism, this catchall designation has happily been relegated to the historic shelf of skeletal pathology.

Solitary unicameral bone cyst occurs mainly in children and adolescents, more often in males, and, with few exceptions, develops in the shaft of a long tubular bone. The upper humeral shaft is its most common site (Fig. 14-33), and the upper femur the next most common (Fig. 14-34), although occasional instances are encountered in the lower femur, the upper or lower tibia, and the forearm bones (Fig. 14-35). Only rarely does one see a bone

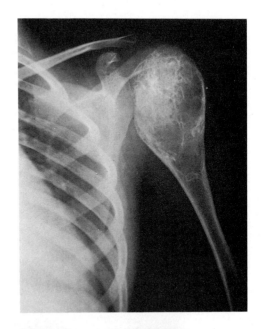

Fig. 14-36. Another unicameral bone cyst in a child, which is unusual in that it involved the entire head of the humerus, as well as the metaphysis. (The epiphyseal cartilage plate is gone.)

A   **B**

Fig. 14-37. **A,** A remarkable bone cyst in the upper metaphysis of the tibia of a 10-year-old child, which also involved the adjacent epiphysis. There was a 2-cm. defect in the epiphyseal cartilage plate at the site of communication between the two fluid-filled compartments. **B,** Follow-up roentgenogram taken 3 years after surgery. The reconstructed, previously cystic area has moved away from the plate.

Fig. 14-38. Photomicrograph of the attenuated wall of a bone cyst. The lining tissue in this instance contained abundant lipid in the form of foam cell aggregates.

cyst elsewhere, such as in a rib, an iliac bone, or a hand or foot bone. It appears to be exceptional also for a unicameral bone cyst to involve the epiphyseal end of the bone, although this may happen (Figs. 14-36 and 14-37).

Pathologically, the lesion is a fluid-containing unicameral cavity. The fluid may be clear and yellow or serosanguineous, particularly if there has been a recent cortical infraction. The overlying cortex is usually thinned and expanded. The periosteal surface is smooth, and there is no new bone apposition unless there has been a pathologic fracture. Its inner (endosteal) surface may show slight ridging and is ordinarily

Fig. 14-39. Roentgenogram of a latent bone cyst in the upper shaft of a humerus, persisting after unsuccessful curettement and packing. The cyst moved away from the plate region but did not heal.

lined by a thin membrane of connective tissue, yielding no more than one or two curettefuls on thorough scraping. Sections of this material may show some new bone formation, blood extravasation, hemosiderin pigment, a scattering of multinuclear macrophages, and often organizing fibrin, which may serve as a substrate for osteoid transformation. Occasionally, especially in older cysts, there may be prominent lipid deposits that take the form of either cholesterol crystals or foam cells containing cholesterol esters (Fig. 14-38).

The evolution of a bone cyst may be seen as developing in two phases: (1) an active phase, in which the lesion in the metaphysis still abuts on the growth plate and is capable of progressive enlargement (Fig. 14-33), and (2) a latent phase, in which the lesion has moved away from the plate down the shaft; the lesion no longer enlarges, but it persists unless it is operated on (Figs. 14-39 and 14-40). The indicated procedure is, of course, thorough curettement and packing with bone chips.[21] Autogenous spongy bone from the iliac crest seems clearly to be the material of choice, although, if this is not available, cancellous bank bone can be utilized. Milled bone is not nearly as satisfactory and the results with Boplant that I have seen have not been encouraging. In any event, it must be recognized that an occasional cyst fails to heal after surgery and may require reoperation or, in a few cases, even a third procedure (Fig. 14-39). Irradiation appears to delay healing and is definitely contraindicated, for this and other reasons.

Fig. 14-40. A, Another latent bone cyst in the upper shaft of a humerus, with a pathologic fracture through its thin cortical wall. **B,** Healing of the fracture shown in **A.** The cyst itself did not disappear.

Pathologic fracture, which often directs attention to the presence of a bone cyst, tends to heal rapidly (Fig. 14-40). While it may be followed by spontaneous healing of the cyst, this happens only occasionally.

The pathogenesis of unicameral bone cyst is still not as well understood as it might be, although it has been the subject of debate and speculation for over 60 years. To be sure, inasmuch as the lesion develops at the epiphyseal plate region, it seems logical to postulate that it has its basis in a local disorder of growth and development. This is begging the question, however—precisely what happens in pathologic terms in the early evolution of a bone cyst is still a matter of conjecture.

Epidermoid cyst in bone

Epidermoid inclusion cysts are relatively unusual in bone and are encountered with any appreciable frequency in only two sites: the calvarium[22] and the tufts of terminal finger phalanges. In the latter site particularly, the possible role of antecedent trauma is sometimes raised as a factor in pathogenesis, but it seems clear that the lesion can develop spontaneously, presumably from an embryonal rest or inclusion.

Epidermoid cysts are characterized radiographically by their sharp outline, as though they had been punched out with a drill press (Fig. 14-41). Pathologically, epidermoid cysts in bone are not essentially different than they are anywhere else.

Aneurysmal bone cyst

Aneurysmal bone cyst is a clinical and pathologic entity that we first became aware of in 1942[20] and later described in a series of papers on the basis of further experience with it.[23-26] The condition is probably more common than is generally realized. Its frequency can be judged from the fact that I was able to survey as many as fifty cases in 1957 (most of which were submitted for consultation), and the tally at present exceeds seventy-five. Undoubtedly, many in-

stances are not identified prior to surgery and, even after tissue examination, some are still mistaken for neoplasm, especially giant cell tumor (Figs. 14-42 and 14-44), sometimes with unfortunate results.

While aneurysmal bone cyst has now been observed in virtually every part of the skeleton, the most common sites are the long bones of the upper and lower extremities and the vertebral column. With reference to age incidence, it is noteworthy that approximately two-thirds of the patients are children or adolescents.

The affected bone site, whatever its location, is completely transformed and ultimately comes to resemble an expanded, blood-filled sponge, which may in time attain impressive size. The communicating pools of venous blood within this reservoir are bordered by a brownish, fibro-osseous meshwork showing microscopically conspicuous giant cell reaction to inordinate vascularity and hemorrhage, as well as fields of osteoid and new bone deposition by way of attempted reconstruction. When such a lesion is explored and the surgeon unroofs its thin expanded dome, he is confronted by blood welling up, though not spurting into the field, which may make thorough curettement difficult.

The roentgenographic picture reflecting these changes is sufficiently distinctive, at least in large limb bones and the vertebral column (the most common sites of localization), to enable one to suspect the condition in the majority of cases, if he is familiar with it.[27] The affected bone area is characteristically expanded, appearing cystically transformed and often eccentrically ballooned-out to a striking degree (Figs. 14-42 to 14-44).

I still adhere to the view that the condition apparently results from some persistent local alteration in hemodynamics leading to increased venous pressure. The anomalous circulation could conceivably result from intraosseous arteriovenous shunts. Radiographic vascular injection studies prior to

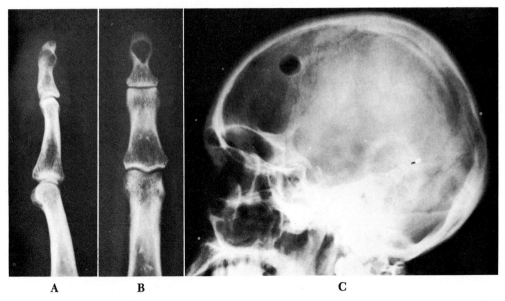

A   B   C

Fig. 14-41. **A** and **B**, Roentgenograms of an epidermoid inclusion cyst in a terminal finger phalanx. There was no history of prior injury. **C**, An epidermoid cyst in the calvarium.

Fig. 14-42. Roentgenogram of an amputated finger ray showing an expanded aneurysmal bone cyst in a metacarpal bone. Radical surgery was done on the mistaken premise that the lesion was a malignant tumor. (Courtesy Armed Forces Medical College, Poona, India.)

Fig. 14-43. Roentgenogram of an aneurysmal bone cyst in the upper metaphysis of the fibula of a 9-year-old boy.

181

Fig. 14-44. Anteroposterior and lateral views of a remarkable aneurysmal bone cyst that originated in a fourth lumbar vertebra (collapsed) and expanded steadily over a period of 5 years, eventually eroding into the duodenum, with fatal exsanguination. At autopsy it was found also to have encroached on the right renal pelvis and encircled the aorta and inferior vena cava. The original biopsy was interpreted as showing a giant cell tumor, and the lesion was said to have been irradiated, but apparently not adequately for effective control. (Courtesy Dr. Tibor Bodi, Jefferson Medical College, Philadelphia.)

surgery with a view to identifying possible abnormal patterns might well be informative and should be done at every opportunity.

The progressive enlargement of an aneurysmal bone cyst can be halted and reconstruction initiated by thorough curettement or roentgen irradiation in moderate dosage. The necessity for *prompt* treatment by whatever means, once the diagnosis is established, must be strongly emphasized. An untreated or poorly treated aneurysmal bone cyst may eventually attain impressive, if not huge, size (Fig. 14-44), sometimes necessitating amputation of a limb,[25] or, in the case of vertebral involvement, resulting in partial destruction of a number of vertebrae[26] and even irreversible paraplegia.

For relatively small or moderately sized lesions in readily accessible sites, curettement and packing with bone chips are calculated to effect a cure and are the treatment of choice. Curettement should be as thorough, however, as the situation will permit, since recurrence is possible otherwise. If irradiation is employed, either as the prime modality or to supplement incomplete eradication by surgical means, previous experience has shown that a total of 1,400 rads should suffice for effective control. Substantially larger doses should be avoided because of the potential hazard of postirradiation sarcoma.[26,28]

In dealing with an aneurysmal bone cyst developing in a vertebral body or its neural arch (such as in the cervical spine of young patients), early diagnosis and appropriate prompt treatment are of the utmost importance. As previously indicated,[26] such lesions, although initially small, may enlarge rapidly and extend to contiguous vertebrae within just a few months, so that the problem of treatment becomes much more formidable. If the changes seen in the roentgenograms suggest aneurysmal bone cyst, prompt conservative biopsy is indicated to confirm this impression. More extensive surgery with a view to substantially complete extirpation is unnecessarily hazardous and should be avoided. As soon as the diagnosis has been established (by a pathologist familiar with the condition), roentgen irradiation in moderate dosage is indicated before the lesion grows much larger. Undue delay or prolonged neglect may have serious consequences (Fig. 14-44).

References

1. Editorial: The Burnett or milk-alkali syndrome, J.A.M.A. **157**:1220, 1955.
2. Pedersen, H. E., and Day, A. J.: Dupuytren's disease of the foot, J.A.M.A. **154**:33, 1954.
3. Pickren, J. W., Smith, A. G., Stevenson, T. W., Jr., and Stout, A. P.: Fibromatosis of the plantar fascia, Cancer **4**:846, 1951.
4. Sutro, C. J.: Slipping of the capital epiphysis of the femur in adolescence, Arch. Surg. **31**:345, 1935.
5. Lacroix, P., and Verbrugge, J.: Slipping of the upper femoral epiphysis: a pathological study, J. Bone Joint Surg. **43-A**:371, 1951.
6. Uhry, E., Jr.: Osgood-Schlatter's disease, Arch. Surg. **48**:406, 1944.
7. LaZerte, G. D., and Rapp, T. H.: Pathogenesis of Osgood-Schlatter's disease, Amer. J. Path. **34**:803, 1958.
8. Sudeck, P.: Arch. Klin. Chir. **62**:147, 1900.
9. Jaffe, H. L.: Bone rarefaction after trauma to large joint regions without fracture, Radiology **33**:305, 1939.
10. Jackson, J. B. J.: A singular case of absorption of bone (a boneless arm), Boston Med. Sci. J. **18**:368, 1838.
11. Case records of Massachusetts General Hospital: Vanishing or disappearing bone disease, New Eng. J. Med. **270**:731, 1964.
12. Gorham, L. W., and Stout, A. P.: Massive osteolysis (acute spontaneous absorption of bone, phantom bone, disappearing bone), J. Bone Joint Surg. **37-A**:985, 1955.
13. Halliday, D. R., Dahlin, D. C., Pugh, D. G., and Young, H. H.: Massive osteolysis and angiomatosis, Radiology **82**:637, 1964.
14. Stern, M. B., and Goldman, R. L.: Disappearing bone disease, Clin. Orthop. **53**:99, 1967.
15. Colonna, P. C.: Spondylolisthesis: analysis of 201 cases, J.A.M.A. **154**:398, 1954.
16. Harris, R. I.: Spondylolisthesis: Hunterian Lecture, Ann. Roy. Coll. Surg. **8**:259, 1951.
17. Gall, E. A., Bennett, C. A., and Bauer, W.: Generalized hypertrophic osteoarthropathy, Amer. J. Path. **27**:349, 1951.
18. Holling, H. E., and Berman, B.: Pulmonary hypertrophic osteoarthropathy, Arch. Intern. Med. **112**:947, 1963.
19. Mendlowitz, M.: Measurements of blood flow and blood pressure in clubbed fingers, J. Clin. Invest. **20**:113, 1941.
20. Jaffe, H. L., and Lichtenstein, L.: Solitary unicameral bone cyst, with emphasis on the roentgen picture, the pathologic appearance and the pathogenesis, Arch. Surg. **44**:1004, 1942.
21. Garceau, G. J., and Gregory, C. F.: Solitary unicameral bone cyst, J. Bone Joint Surg. **36-A**:267, 1954.
22. Kleinsasser, O., and Albrecht, H.: Die Epidermoide der Schädelknochen, Langenbeck. Arch. Klin. Chir. **285**:498, 1957.
23. Jaffe, H. L.: Aneurysmal bone cyst, Bull. Hosp. Joint Dis. **11**:3, 1950.
24. Lichtenstein, L.: Aneurysmal bone cyst: a pathological entity commonly mistaken for giant-cell tumor and occasionally for hemangioma and osteogenic sarcoma, Cancer **3**:279, 1950.
25. Lichtenstein, L.: Aneurysmal bone cyst: further observations, Cancer **6**:1228, 1953.
26. Lichtenstein, L.: Aneurysmal bone cyst: observations on fifty cases, J. Bone Joint Surg. **39-A**:873, 1957.
27. Sherman, R. S., and Soong, K. Y.: Radiology **68**:54, 1957.
28. Dahlin, D. C., Besse, B. E., Jr., Pugh, D. G., and Ghormley, R. K.: Aneurysmal bone cyst, Radiology **64**:56, 1955.

Chapter 15

Disorders of synovial joints

The linings of synovial joints are very labile and react to a wide variety of changes and noxious influences originating locally or elsewhere in the body. In its response, the multipotent capacity of the synovium becomes evident. Quite apart from the usual manifestations of response to injury, the lining cells can multiply and become several or many layers in thickness; they can phagocytose hemosiderin and lipid, urates and ochronotic pigment, and bacteria and foreign particles; they can give rise to histiocytes (or macrophages) in response to infection, rheumatoid inflammation, and pigmented villonodular synovitis; they can give rise to fibroblasts, resulting in synovial or subsynovial scarring; and they can elaborate a mucinous fluid rich in hyaluronic acid, excess of which leads to effusion or hydrarthrosis. In addition, the synovium is capable of forming cartilagenous and osseous bodies by metaplasia, as in osteochondromatosis. On occasion, it may undergo neoplastic change, giving rise to synovial sarcoma and even synovial chondrosarcoma.

The articular cartilages, too, are vulnerable to trauma, degeneration (as in osteoarthritis), prolonged hemarthrosis (as in hemophilia), changes in certain metabolic disorders (gout, hereditary ochronosis), infections, overgrowth by inflammatory pannus (as in rheumatoid arthirtis), and injury from whatever cause initiates a sequence of events that will be indicated presently.

The articular bone ends (within the joint capsule) may be involved initially by infection (osteomyelitis or tuberculosis spreading to the capsule), bone infarcts (especially in the hip, leading to subsequent arthritic changes), lipid storage (as in Gaucher's disease), and so on. More often, though, they become implicated secondarily in the familiar changes of osteoarthritis, as a sequel of some process that damages or destroys the articular cartilage.

The discussion that follows will attempt in an orderly sequence to indicate the basic pathologic changes that ensue in the more common disorders of joints and in some that are more unusual. A number of these conditions have already been discussed in other chapters and will be mentioned again only briefly for the sake of completeness. The clinical background of each of these disorders will be considered insofar as it appears essential for clear definition or orientation.

Chronic villous nonspecific synovitis

Chronic villous nonspecific synovitis is a descriptive designation commonly used by pathologists for the nonspecific reaction of the synovial lining of a joint, such as a knee, to a wide variety of irritating factors. It may be induced by anything that causes internal derangement of a joint and it is

Fig. 15-1. Photomicrograph showing the changes commonly observed in chronic villous nonspecific synovitis.

Fig. 15-2. Instance of chronic villous synovitis in which the inflammation is more intense than in Fig. 15-1. In the absence of abundant fibrinoid exudate, this picture should not be interpreted as necessarily suggesting rheumatoid disease.

185

Fig. 15-3. Photomicrograph showing focal injury to an articular cartilage surface and its organization by granulation tissue.

therefore observed frequently in routine orthopedic surgical specimens. It is sometimes seen in children with capsular thickening and arthralgia, especially after enteric infections. It may also be seen at times in women at menopause, in which case there may be remission after estrogen therapy. In some instances, trauma may be a factor. In still others, no predisposing factor can be implicated.

Whatever the cause of the reaction, one observes a varying degree of villous hypertrophy (this is the only way in which the synovium can expand or enlarge). Usually associated with it is slight thickening of the lining, capillary vascularization, a sprinkling of chronic inflammatory cells, and slight synovial or subsynovial fibrosis (Fig. 15-1). At times, the inflammatory reaction may be more intense, even with the formation of focal nodular aggregates, without this necessarily implying rheumatoid etiology (Fig. 15-2).

Joint changes following trauma

Intraarticular fractures frequently injure the articular cartilage as well as the joint capsule. When there is comminution of the bone, compression with telescoping, or dislocation with extensive tearing of ligaments so that protracted immobilization is required, fibrous ankylosis with pain and loss of motion and sometimes even bony ankylosis may be the end result.

Trauma to joints without fracture may likewise induce certain deleterious effects in the articular capsule. The articular cartilage may be injured in one or more areas; while the defects are slowly repaired, they are filled with fibrous connective tissue rather than regenerated hyaline cartilage (Fig. 15-3). A number of changes may also be observed in the synovium, namely, some thickening of the lining, villous hypertrophy, fibrosis, slight fibrin exudate at times, possibly occasional nests of foam cells, and discoloration of the lining (to yellow-brown or darker brown) by hemosiderin pigment resulting from hemorrhage. Actually, it takes surprisingly little hemosiderin to impart gross coloration to the lining. When there is abundant hemosiderin deposition, pathologists sometimes consider the possibility of pigmented villonodular synovitis, although the essential component of active histiocytic proliferation is lacking.

Altogether, the synovial changes described are usually not specific enough in themselves to justify a diagnosis of *post-traumatic synovitis* (or arthritis), it seems to me, although one may suspect that they result from an injury, particularly when the latter is well documented.

Injury to joint regions may also cause the formation of *joint bodies,* whose long-

Fig. 15-4. A joint body composed entirely of cartilage that has become calcified. On its surface (particularly at the left), one sees successive layers of cartilage formed by accretion.

Fig. 15-5. An osteochondral joint body (from a knee) presenting a necrotic osseous core and a cartilage periphery, which has increased in thickness from the deposition of successive layers of cartilage. A "joint mouse" such as this could conceivably represent a broken-off marginal osteophyte or an old osteoarticular fracture fragment.

187

term effect is to favor articular damage (like foreign bodies in a closed gearbox). Such "joint mice" may represent detached bits of articular cartilage, or small osteo-articular fracture fragments, or marginal osteophytes. To be sure, there are other sources of joint bodies—osteochondromatosis of the synovium or a focus of osteochondritis dissecans of the knee that has become free—but we are not concerned with these at the moment.

Whatever the origin of joint bodies, they are nourished by the synovial fluid and grow slowly by the accretion of layers of cartilage on their surface. Eventually, they may become several or many times their original size. The cartilage component can become calcified, but ossification does not occur, since this would require a blood supply (Figs. 15-4 and 15-5).

Infections of joints

Infections of joints, on the whole, are of distinctly varied nature and may be associated with sepsis, tuberculosis, syphilis, mycoses (especially coccidiomycosis), and even certain viral infections. Many aspects of joint infection have already been considered in Chapter 3 and will not be reiterated here. As previously indicated, it is often difficult, if not impossible, to draw a sharp line of demarcation between infections of bone and those of joints, inasmuch as the two are frequently associated. Also mentioned briefly will be certain conditions of as yet undetermined etiology, such as sarcoid and Reiter's disease, since there is a strong clinical presumption that they are of infectious nature.

Pyogenic arthritis (septic arthritis; acute infectious arthritis; suppurative arthritis; pyarthrosis). Pyogenic arthritis, which is usually monarticular, is most often associated with bacteremia or with irruption of a focus of infection in bone into a neighboring joint. Occasionally, it may be a complication of penetrating wounds or joint surgery or of intraarticular injections or as-piration. As in osteomyelitis, the major pathogenic microorganisms are *Staphylococcus aureus* and *Streptococcus hemolyticus,* although occasionally *Gonococcus, Meningococcus, Diplococcus pneumoniae, Haemophilus influenzae, Brucella,* and still others may be responsible for joint infection. While the widespread use of antibiotics has sharply reduced the incidence of pyarthrosis, it may still be a problem in vulnerable premature infants, in those on prolonged massive steroid therapy, in cancer patients receiving marrow-depressing chemotherapeutic agents predisposing to unusual infections, and in patients infected with resistant strains of staphylococci.

The affected joint is usually red, hot, swollen, and very tender. Constitutionally, as one might expect, there is associated fever, leukocytosis, and elevated sedimentation rate. The situation calls for prompt blood culture, as well as culture of aspirated synovial fluid or pus, and bacterial sensitivity studies. Penicillin or tetracycline may well be the antibiotic of choice, although others are often required when dealing with resistant strains of staphylococci. In any event, systemic therapy is usually indicated, in addition to local aspiration, irrigation, and instillation of antibiotic agents. These measures apparently have largely obviated the necessity for incision and drainage, which were once common practice.

The synovial lining of the infected joint capsule is edematous, hyperemic, and acutely inflamed (Fig. 15-6). Apart from this, the tendency to rapid lysis of the articular cartilage by the proteolytic enzymes of pus cells is of paramount importance and underscores the necessity for early diagnosis and treatment if one is to avoid serious damage to the articular bone ends and bony ankylosis. With staphylococcal infection particularly, destruction of cartilage may ensue rapidly. Some of the most solidly fused joints I have ever seen have been the result of healed staphylo-

Fig. 15-6. Photomicrograph of the synovial lining of a knee joint infected by *Streptococcus hemolyticus*, showing marked edema, engorgement of blood vessels, and intense inflammatory exudate. Most of the inflammatory cells are polymorphonuclear leukocytes.

coccal pyarthrosis in the preantibiotic era. Other possible complications of untreated or poorly treated severe pyogenic arthritis, now fortunately uncommon, are rupture of abscess into extracapsular soft parts, extension of infection into the articular bone ends, infarction of bone from interference with blood supply (in a femoral head, for example), and, in children, dislocation and epiphyseal separation.

Gonococcal arthritis deserves special mention here, although the effectiveness of penicillin in treating the primary infection of the urethra or cervix has sharply reduced its incidence. In untreated or resistant cases, after a latent period of some 2 to 4 weeks, severe manifestations of arthritis may suddenly appear. Initial polyarthralgia is soon followed by localizing signs in one joint, usually the knee, hip, ankle, or wrist. Gono-

cocci can often be cultured from the joint fluid or exudate, but even if they are not, penicillin in large doses should be administered systemically in addition to appropriate local therapy. Here again, one must stress the importance of effective early treatment in view of the hazards of serious damage to articular cartilage surfaces and of extensive bone atrophy.

Tuberculosis of joints. Apart from spondylitis (with caseation, gibbus, paravertebral cold abscess, and possibly spinal cord compression), one of the more common expressions of skeletal involvement by tuberculosis is arthritis. The knee joint is most often involved in adults and the hip in children, although occasionally the shoulder, elbow, wrist, or some other joint may be affected. The onset of infection is usually insidious, and the course generally indolent

Fig. 15-7. Photomicrograph showing spread of tuberculous granulation tissue beneath articular cartilage, which is substantially necrotic and in the process of being sequestrated.

and protracted, leading to progressive destruction of the capsule and articular bone ends, unless the disease is controlled by specific chemotherapy, immobilization, and surgery, when indicated.

Arthritis of long standing affecting a single joint must be presumed to be tuberculous until proved otherwise. A positive tuberculin skin test indicates exposure and hypersensitivity essentially and in itself is not conclusive. The roentgenographic changes, while helpful, may be varied and unusual and, by the same token, are not infallible. For that matter, frozen section of a synovial biopsy is not always dependable either, because of the random distribution of tubercle. However, a firm diagnosis may often be established preoperatively by culture and/or guinea pig inoculation of aspirated synovial fluid. The latter is likely to show a low total white cell count, few pus cells, a low sugar concentration, and high protein content.

While tuberculous lesions in joints may start in the synovium, they usually begin in one or both osteoarticular bone ends. In the latter event, there is a tendency for tuberculous granulation tissue sooner or later to dissect beneath the articular cartilage, which becomes necrotic, softened, and uplifted (Fig. 15-7). Spread of infection over the synovial lining leads to effusion, relatively abundant fibrin exudate, and the development of tuberculous granulation tissue (Fig. 15-8, *A*). Eventually, if the process is not checked, one may see thickening and induration of the capsule and periarticular soft tissues (Fig. 15-8, *B*), burrowing fistulae, and extensive secondary destruction of bone, with irreparable damage to the function of the joint as a whole. As previously indicated, arthrodesis may well be the surgical treatment of choice for badly damaged weight-bearing joints.

Coccidiomycosis of joints. The subject of skeletal coccidiomycosis in general

Fig. 15-8. **A,** Tuberculous synovitis of a knee joint, showing fibrin exudate on the lining surface and chronically inflamed granulation tissue containing a number of tubercles. **B,** Another photomicrograph showing tuberculous reaction in the wall of a subdeltoid bursa.

Fig. 15-9. Photomicrograph of a skeletal lesion of coccidiomycosis showing acute inflammation and necrosis (on the left), as well as histiocytic response and the formation of a tubercle-like nodule containing a doubly refractile spherule of *Coccidioides immitis.*

has been discussed previously (Chapter 3). As for joint involvement specifically, two relevant observations may be cited here. The manifestation of "desert rheumatism" —the development of transient painful, tender, and slightly swollen joints in the course of primary pulmonary disease, often associated with erythema nodosum—is well known in endemic areas. This would seem to be a manifestation of hypersensitivity.

What is perhaps not common knowledge is that there may be chronic indolent involvement of a single joint lasting for years, without clinically demonstrable disease elsewhere.[1] The affected joint is likely to be swollen and painful, with some limitation of motion. Prior to tissue examination the condition may simulate tuberculous arthritis. I have seen material from at least four cases in point; in three a knee joint was af-

fected and in another an ankle (Fig. 15-9). In one such instance, in which the tissue reaction closely resembled that of tuberculosis, it was only after a persistent search that a single spherule of *Coccidioides immitis* was found within a giant cell in a granulomatous tubercle-like nodule. In the matter of treatment, amphotericin B is the antibiotic currently used, but it is not always as effective as it might be.

Joint manifestations in syphilis. In congenital lues, osteochondritis appearing at or soon after birth may be responsible for joint disability. Involvement of the upper humeral epiphysis, for example, can result in flaccidity of the arm (Parrot's pseudoparalysis). In older children (between the ages of 8 and 16 years), a painless bilateral synovitis of the knee may sometimes develop (Clutton's joints) in association with keratitis, periostitis, and other manifestations.

During the secondary stage of acquired syphilis, painful swollen joints (suggesting rheumatoid arthritis) may occasionally appear, but this too is an infrequent manifestation. By all odds the most common joint disorder is that encountered in tertiary syphilis, namely, the Charcot joint, the neurotrophic changes of which result from dorsal column sclerosis in the spinal cord, as seen in tabes. The pathogenesis and evolution of these changes have already been described in Chapter 9.

Joint manifestations in viral diseases. In the area of viral disease, there is more clinical speculation available than hard pathologic fact. While arthralgias are common in influenza and epidemic viral arthritis[2] and an occasional feature of other viral infections, little if anything is known apparently about their synovial reflection. Perhaps this is because the pathologist does not ordinarily examine the joints at autopsy when the opportunity arises, even though the sternoclavicular joint and the knee are readily accessible.

The development of migratory polyarthralgias and arthritis some 2 weeks after mumps parotitis (and orchitis) has been well documented clinically.[3,4] In rubella, a synovial mononuclear reaction has been noted on biopsy,[5] but there is apparently no record of examination of an entire involved joint. Joint infection has also been observed as an unusual complication of chickenpox, but this is apparently of secondary pyogenic nature.

Reiter's syndrome. Arthritis is a feature of Reiter's syndrome, along with urethritis, conjunctivitis, and, often, a peculiar dermatitis as well. While its etiology is not clear, a strong suspicion of some infectious agent prevails (pleuropneumonia-like organisms, mycoplasma, and *Bedsonia* have been implicated). It is for that reason that the disease is tentatively considered here under the head of joint infections.

Usually a number of joints are affected, particularly the knees and ankles, although occasionally only a single joint may be involved. Inflammatory changes in the heel cord are also common. The pathologic changes in the synovium have been described[6] as those of chronic nonspecific inflammation with a lymphocytic and plasma cell infiltrate. While the arthritic condition is usually self-limited, it may recur and sometimes becomes chronic. In the latter event, the late roentgenographic changes are indicative of cartilage damage and the development of secondary osteoarthritis. Curiously enough, occasional cases are said to progress to true rheumatoid arthritis or ankylosing spondylitis.[6] This observation, along with reports of cardiac complications and the favorable response to steroid therapy, would suggest that the syndrome may conceivably be a peculiar expression of rheumatic disease.

Joint involvement in sarcoidosis (Besnier-Boeck-Schaumann's disease). While the etiology of sarcoidosis is still uncertain, it is mentioned here for want of a better place to categorize it. Sokoloff and Bunim,[7] in reporting on five cases proved by synovial biopsy in which polyarthritis was a conspicuous specific feature, point out that joint involvement in sarcoid disease may be more common than is generally realized. Some instances in point may be mistaken for rheumatoid arthritis or rheumatic fever. Their article is valuable also for its bibliography.

As previously mentioned (Chapter 14), extensive regional involvement of tendon sheaths may also occur as an unusual major manifestation of sarcoidosis.

Joint damage resulting from chronic hemarthrosis

While a single hemorrhage into a joint can be resorbed readily, leaving only light hemosiderin staining of the synovial lining as a residuum, repeated, long-term hemarthrosis (or hemosiderosis) from whatever cause can have deleterious effects. That it may lead to serious permanent damage to

Fig. 15-10. A, Photomicrograph showing partially calcified urate deposits within the synovial lining of the knee joint of a patient with moderately severe gout. **B,** From the surface of a patella in a case of gout, showing a urate-containing connective tissue pannus over the modified articular cartilage.

small and large joints in untreated hemophilia and hemophilia-like conditions has already been indicated (Chapter 10). It may also be a factor in diffuse pigmented villonodular synovitis of the knee joint, and occasionally other joints, if the condition is allowed to continue long enough without effective therapy, be it synovectomy or irradiation. In advanced or terminal hemochromatosis, one may find joint effusion in the knee, for example, as well as obvious brown hemosiderin-staining of the articular cartilage and synovium.[8,9] In scurvy, as previously noted (Chapter 4), painful hemor-

Fig. 15-11. **A,** Drawing showing the striking changes of ochronotic arthritis in a knee joint. (Courtesy Dr. E. Mathias.) **B,** Photomicrograph of a section of synovium of a knee joint in a case of hereditary ochronosis showing numerous fragments of broken-off, heavily pigmented articular cartilage ground into the synovial lining and the sublining tissues.

rhages occur within and about the joints, among many other sites, although these are usually overshadowed by the lesions in the epiphyses of limb bones. Finally, one may occasionally see comparable hemorrhages about a joint or even into the joint itself (such as a knee or an elbow) in severe purpura (hemorrhagic arthritis or arthritic purpura).

It would appear that injury to the articular cartilage in these circumstances results from a number of contributing factors. Impregnation of the cartilage by blood pigment is apparently harmful in itself. In experimental hemarthrosis of comparatively long standing, it has been shown by electron microscopy that iron-containing bodies are deposited in chondrocytes and that this may be associated with intracellular degeneration.[10] It seems reasonable to postulate also that the addition of substantial amounts of blood or its derivatives to the synovial fluid may well interfere with adequate nutrition of the articular cartilage. Still another factor to be considered is overgrowth of the articular cartilage by the folds of the brownishly discolored synovial membrane, which, in time, undergoes matting from extensive villous hypertrophy.

Arthritic manifestations of certain metabolic disorders

We are concerned here specifically with gout, hereditary ochronosis, and (indirectly) Gaucher's disease. The skeletal alterations in general of these inborn errors of metabolism have already been discussed (Chapter 6), and the observations made will not be reiterated here. A number of illustrative photomicrographs have been introduced, however, to highlight the joint changes, particularly in chronic tophaceous gout and in ochronosis (Figs. 15-10 and 15-11).

Neurotrophic joint disorders

The skeletal changes that may occur in neurotrophic disorders, of which tabes dorsalis and syringomyelia are the most common, have already been considered in Chapter 9.

Osteoarthritis

Osteoarthritis (degenerative arthritis, degenerative joint disease, senescent arthritis, hypertrophic arthritis, arthritis deformans, osteoarthrosis) is by all odds the most common expression of arthritic change. It is characterized pathologically by degenerative alterations in the articular cartilages. This is eventually combined with hypertrophic changes in the bone ends, leading to deformation of the articular surfaces. Inflammatory reaction in the synovial membrane, so conspicuous in rheumatoid arthritis, is usually insignificant.

The alterations in the articular cartilage may reflect primary degenerative or senescent change, or they may follow in the wake of damage to the articular cartilages from other causes (secondary hypertrophic arthritis), such as previous infection or trauma with intraarticular fracture (Figs. 15-12 to 15-16). In the hip joint, for example, slipped epiphysis, Perthes' disease, Gaucher's disease, or caisson disease may be significant initiating factors; in the knee, "joint mice," osteochondritis dissecans, osteochondromatosis, or torn menisci of long standing may be responsible.

Whatever its basis, the primary change in osteoarthritis is in the articular cartilage, which becomes yellowish, fibrillized, nappy, rubbed down, or denuded (Fig. 15-12). The nature of the yellow (or yellow-brown) senescent pigmentation in biochemical terms has been investigated, but it is not yet fully understood.[11] Increased wear and tear through weight-bearing and excessive or abnormal use of a joint is known to accelerate the tendency to degenerative changes, but the latter may be observed at times in comparatively young adults, in so-called chondromalacia of the patella, for example (Fig. 15-12).

Where the cartilage is denuded and blood vessels reach the surface, there is a

A   B

Fig. 15-12. **A,** Photograph of articular surface of a patella showing flaking and fibrillization of the cartilage, as seen in so-called chondromalacia of the patella. The linear horizontal depression apparently resulted from an injury. (The patient also had a bucket-handle tear of a meniscus.) **B,** Low power photomicrograph of a specimen of chondromalacia of the patella showing fraying and degeneration of its articular surface (reflected in a yellowish nap in the gross).

localized advance in the line of ossification. Marginal exostoses (osteophytes) develop, usually around the periphery. When the latter are well established, they may cause extensive deformity of the articular bone ends, pain, and limitation of motion. The central contact surfaces tend to become eburnated and often highly polished, like the surface of a billiard ball. The synovium, quite understandably, becomes thickened and modified as a result of chronic irritation; but, as noted, there is no real inflammation, as there is in rheumatoid arthritis (Fig. 15-15), nor do the muscles undergo atrophy. What happens to the subchondral bone depends on whether there is motion in the affected joint: if there has been some motion, the subchondral bone tends to become sclerotic; if there is no appreciable motion, the bone undergoes atrophy. Foci of fibrous tissue may develop in the subchondral bone, and these can undergo degeneration and cystic softening (Fig. 15-14), appearing as cyst-like rarefactions in roentgenograms (if they become large enough to be visualized).

This sequence of events may be observed in the large mushroomed femoral head of osteoarthritis of the hip (malum coxae senilis); in spondylosis deformans, when the vertebral bodies are fused by exostoses ex-

Fig. 15-13. Photomicrograph showing degeneration and erosion of articular cartilage, as seen in osteoarthritis.

Fig. 15-14. Another section showing the changes of osteoarthritis. The articular cartilage is extensively degenerated and frayed (in other areas, it was eroded down to the bone). Within the thickened subchondral bone, one sees fibrous connective tissue that has undergone cystic softening.

Fig. 15-15. Section of the synovial lining of a knee joint in a case of osteoarthritis. There are two bits of articular cartilage embedded in it, and around them, some fibrosis and chronic irritative reaction. Note, however, that the lining is not hyperplastic and that there is no fibrinoid exudate, such as one might expect in rheumatoid synovitis.

Fig. 15-16. Photograph (reduced) showing changes of severe osteoarthritis in a knee of a patient who 50 years previously had fallen down an elevator shaft. The smaller bodies on the right represent old modified osteoarticular fracture fragments.

tending across the intervertebral disks; in Heberden's nodes, reflecting marginal exostoses about the terminal interphalangeal joints; and in many other comparable situations.

Rheumatoid arthritis

Rheumatoid arthritis (atrophic arthritis, ankylosing arthritis, proliferative arthritis) is a major member of a group of inflammatory systemic connective tissue diseases ("collagen" diseases), which also includes rheumatic fever, disseminated lupus erythematosus, periarteritis nodosa (polyarteritis), dermatomyositis, systemic sclerosis (scleroderma), and possibly other conditions.

While the target sites vary in these disorders, to be sure, in their pathologic reaction they exhibit certain features in common: namely, swelling and modification of the ground substance, fibrinoid degeneration or necrosis, fibroblastic proliferation, and a predominantly mononuclear inflammatory response. It has been suggested that this response may reflect altered immune reactions, and this area is a subject of active investigation.[12,13] In some of the disorders at least, a tissue hypersensitivity reaction to specific agents can be logically postulated, as in the case of rheumatic fever and certain forms of periarteritis nodosa, as indeed Klinge indicated back in the early 1930's. Furthermore, the observation of occasional cases with overlapping clinical and pathologic manifestations referable to two or more of the systemic connective tissue diseases would suggest that the latter have certain pathogenetic factors in common.

In rheumatoid arthritis, the linings of the synovial joints are the principal target site, although tendon sheaths and bursal sacs may also be affected, as well as the eye, lungs, pleura, heart, and occasionally other visceral sites. Also, subcutaneous rheumatoid nodules develop at one time or another in some 20% of all cases. We are concerned here primarily with the inflammatory joint lesions and especially with the pathologic changes. The clinical picture is well known from countless articles and monographs and hardly needs exposition.

Commonly, there is multiple joint involvement, but there are undoubtedly some cases in which apparently only a single joint is affected, clinically at least. Joints of the hands and feet are involved most often, but many others in both upper and lower extremities and in the vertebral column are commonly implicated. Whatever the site, the process starts as a synovitis (in contrast to osteoarthritis, in which the initial lesion is damage to the articular cartilage). Later, there is extension of inflammatory pannus over the articular cartilages (Fig. 15-17), and eventually loss of function and often severe and disabling deformity.

The roentgenographic alterations parallel and reflect the pathologic changes. The early manifestations are those of soft tissue swelling, thickening of the affected joint capsule, and significant osteoporosis unrelated to steroid therapy and presumably resulting from disuse and perhaps inflammatory hyperemia. Later, destruction of articular cartilage is reflected in narrowing of the joint space and, with the advent of secondary osteoarthritis following in the wake of denudation of cartilage, in such changes as marginal osteophytes and small subchondral rarefactions. In the late stage of severe disease, one may eventually see subluxation, flexion contracture, ankylosis, and other deformities (Fig. 15-18). In a terminal, burned-out stage (as seen in joint specimens obtained at autopsy) it may be difficult to distinguish clearly the sequelae of earlier rheumatoid arthritis from the heavy overlay of secondary osteoarthritis after the inflammatory reaction has subsided. In these circumstances, one must have recourse to a good clinical history to determine the probable sequence of events.

The pathologic picture of the synovitis varies somewhat, depending on the stage of the disease at the time of examination. The inflammation may be subacute or more

Fig. 15-17. Photomicrograph of an articular bone end in rheumatoid arthritis showing extension of vascularized, inflammatory pannus containing abundant fibrinoid exudate (dark staining) over the damaged and disappearing articular cartilage.

| A | B | C |

Fig. 15-18. Roentgenograms from well-established cases of rheumatoid arthritis affecting the knee, elbow, and wrist joints respectively and showing distinct narrowing of the joint space (reflecting loss of articular cartilage), osteoporosis, and evidence of secondary osteoarthritis.

chronic. In general, the synovium is thickened and congested and shows villous hypertrophy, extensive fibrinoid deposits on the lining, and infiltration of the synovium and sublining connective tissue by large numbers of inflammatory cells, sometimes clumped in aggregates. These inflammatory cells are mainly lymphocytes, macrophages (of synovial origin), and plasma cells. If the joint is "hot" at the time of synovectomy or biopsy, there may also be a sprinkling of polymorphonuclear leukocytes. The plasma cells contain abundant cytoplasmic ribonucleic acid, which reacts with methyl green–pyronin to produce a deep, red-purple color.[14] These are also the cells that are

Fig. 15-19. Photomicrographs of the synovial lining of the knee joint from two cases of clinical rheumatoid arthritis showing intense villous synovitis.

rich in immune globulins; this can be demonstrated by appropriate immunofluorescent techniques.

It should be emphasized that none of the features of the inflammatory reaction are specific in themselves, since one may find them in other conditions. As for fibrinoid deposits (and "rice" bodies) in particular, they are by no means peculiar to rheumatoid lesions. They are seen with regularity not only in tuberculous synovitis but also in ordinary, chronically irritated bursae. What is helpful is the composite picture, particularly the intensity of the reaction. In most situations, the pathologist is well advised to state simply that the reaction observed microscopically is consistent with rheumatoid arthritis, if such is the case, implying that the diagnosis must be based upon clinical evidence as well (Fig. 15-19). For that matter, the demonstration of "rheumatoid factor" (gamma globulin) by a variety of laboratory techniques, while helpful, is not specific. This is true also of examination of aspirated synovial fluid.

The subcutaneous nodule is said to be pathognomonic for rheumatoid arthritis, although a comparable lesion may also occur in rheumatic fever. They develop most often in the elbow region, the olecranon bursa, the knee region, and the tendon sheaths of fingers and toes but may also be encountered elsewhere. In the early stage of its development, as Sokoloff and his associates[15] indicated, the appearance of vascular granulation tissue is a prominent feature, and the blood vessels may show inflammatory changes and occasionally even necrosis. In routine surgical specimens, however, these changes are not usually observed. The familiar conventional picture is that of a serpiginous focus of collagen necrosis, bordered by palisaded histiocytes and macrophages (Fig. 15-20). It should be noted also that in autopsied subjects with long-standing but still active rheumatoid arthritis, one

Fig. 15-20. Rheumatoid nodule within vascularized, collagenous connective tissue (elbow region).

may occasionally observe similar granulomas in visceral sites, such as the pleura, lungs, heart, or dura.

The skeletal muscles in the vicinity of affected joints tend to undergo atrophy and wasting. Focal lymphocytic infiltrates have been found in them (as well as in the sheaths of large peripheral nerves), but one must be wary of ascribing any specificity to them, inasmuch as collections of mononuclear cells may be found in muscle tissue in a wide variety of orthopedic conditions unrelated to rheumatoid arthritis.

Attention may also be directed here to two other relevant pathologic observations of significance. First, in Great Britain at least, rheumatoid arthritis is the most common cause of amyloidosis at the present time.[14] This ties in well with the concept of an altered immune reaction featuring the formation of abnormal globulins. Second, the repeated intraarticular therapeutic injection of cortisone or hydrocortisone entails a distinct hazard, since it may be followed by accelerated joint destruction, sometimes so extensive as to suggest Charcot arthropathy[16] (although no neurologic disease is present). The pathogenesis of this curious phenomenon is not well understood.

"Rheumatoid" spondylitis (ankylosing spondylitis, Marie-Strümpell arthritis, von Bechterew's arthritis, spondylitis rhizomelic, pelvospondylitis ossificans[17]) is often classified as a special manifestation of rheumatoid arthritis, although there is still apparently some uncertainty about the correctness of this view. It is true that some 20% of these patients present changes in peripheral joints resembling those seen in rheumatoid arthritis. On the other hand, there are dissimilar features: the predilection for males, its familial incidence at times, the rarity of subcutaneous nodules, the beneficial response to roentgen therapy, and the negative agglutination tests. Be that as it may, the intervertebral articulations show fibrous or bony ankylosis with osseous bridges between the bodies. These changes, together with demineralization of the vertebral bodies and calcification of the lateral spinal ligaments, are eventually reflected in the picture of the "bamboo spine" or the "poker back," which may require corrective osteotomy for improved function.

Still's disease (juvenile rheumatoid arthritis) is a chronic progressive polyarthritis in children, usually below the age of 10 years, associated with generalized lymphadenopathy (inguinal, axillary, cervical, epitrochlear) and, often fever, secondary anemia, and splenomegaly. Cutaneous symptoms are prominent in some patients who may manifest frequent attacks of urticaria or erythema and sometimes erythema multiforme. The arthritic changes resemble those in rheumatoid arthritis of adults. The joints are usually symmetrically involved and many joints may be affected, particularly shoulders, elbows, wrists, fingers, knees, and feet, and occasionally the vertebral column (cervical), the jaw (temporomandibular joint), and the sternoclavicular articulation. Some of the earliest and most severely affected joints may be the proximal interphalangeal joints of the fingers. The clinical course is usually progressive for months and sometimes years. While crippling may ensue, spontaneous remission and substantial recovery are not unusual.

Felty's syndrome (rheumatoid arthritis with hypersplenism) is an old designation for rheumatoid arthritis in adults associated with splenomegaly and leukopenia. These patients usually have severe arthritic manifestations.

Association of rheumatoid arthritis with psoriasis. While it may be coincidental, in certain patients (approximately 3%) with severe rheumatoid arthritis there appears to be a peculiar, more intimate relationship designated as *"psoriatic arthritis."* In such patients the exacerbations and remissions of the two diseases are likely to coincide, the distal interphalangeal joints are involved, and there is roentgenographic evidence of resorption of bone at the articular margins.

Joint manifestations in other systemic connective tissue diseases

More clinical observations than informative pathologic data are available in the area of systemic connective tissue diseases. There is definitely a need for more synovial biopsies in relevant cases and for the pathologist who has an unusual opportunity to perform an autopsy in any of these diseases to examine as many joints as possible and to obtain specimens of synovium for microscopic examination.

Rheumatic fever. Rheumatic fever, an acute or chronic inflammatory disease, is initiated by a preceding group A hemolytic streptococcal infection. It has also been induced by streptococcal vaccination (type 3 streptococcal M protein) in healthy siblings of patients with rheumatic fever.[18] In this connection also, one may recall the old animal experiments of Rich and Gregory[19] indicating that lesions having the basic characteristics of rheumatic carditis can result from anaphylactic hypersensitivity. Be that as it may, clinical rheumatic fever affects not only synovial joints but also the heart (pancarditis), the meninges (chorea), and possibly other connective tissue structures. As noted, subcutaneous nodules are also observed, as is erythema marginatum. There is apparently an important familial factor. While its peak incidence is in children above the age of 5 years, there is said to be an appreciable incidence in adults.

The joint manifestations, while acute in onset, are usually not severe, and the number of joints involved is generally small. Those most frequently affected are the ankles, knees, small joints of the foot, wrists, or elbows, and they are usually attacked in succession rather than simultaneously. Sometimes the symptoms are limited to a single joint, such as a hip, knee, or ankle. At times, they are less in the joints themselves than in the periarticular tissues and muscles,

so that they are dismissed as "growing pains."

As for the pathologic changes in affected joints, there is seldom an opportunity to examine them in the stage of acute inflammation. I have not had occasion to see any relevant specimens at first hand, and the casual statements found in texts are too vague to be very informative.

Disseminated lupus erythematosus. Among the many other protean manifestations of lupus erythematosis, joint involvement is noted in more than 75% of patients. The arthralgias, however, are likely to be migratory, so that permanent clinical or roentgenographic evidence of arthritis is said to be found in only 35% of patients. Here again, one is handicapped by the paucity of available material. The pathologic nature of these arthritic changes apparently needs clarification.

The arthritis of systemic lupus erythematosus is held by some to be different from that of rheumatoid arthritis, although this is disputed.[20] According to Gardner,[14] the cellular synovial reaction is less intense, but more fibrinoid exudate is likely to be present.

Dermatomyositis. Among the varied manifestations of dermatomyositis, those referable to the joints and muscles are noteworthy here. Arthralgias are mild, and the pathologic changes that they reflect are apparently not well understood, although Aegerter and Kirkpatrick[21] state (without offering supporting evidence) that they resemble those of mild rheumatoid arthritis. Involved muscles may undergo marked degeneration and atrophy, and joint deformities from flexion contractures develop late in the disease.

Scleroderma. Among the skeletal changes in scleroderma that may be cited are sclerodactyly and Raynaud's phenomenon, sometimes associated with calcinosis of the skin (Fig. 14-8). Arthralgias are less frequent, but the tightening of the skin that ensues may eventually result in diminished joint

205

motion. Certain dental changes have been described, particularly widening of the periodontal space, disappearance of the lamina dura, and, occasionally, loosening of teeth.

Periarteritis nodosa (polyarteritis). As noted, some cases of polyarteritis may be triggered by hypersensitivity reaction to numerous drugs and other substances. The essential pathologic lesion is that of focal inflammation and necrosis of small and medium-sized arteries throughout the body. Skeletal muscle lesions are quite common, and biopsy of an affected muscle may serve to establish a diagnosis, although random sampling may not be rewarding. Arthritis is a very unusual manifestation, although arthralgias associated with polyneuritis and myositis are not infrequently observed.

Some remarks on the classification and pathology of nonarticular "rheumatism"

It has been stated[22] that some 25% of patients seeking help ostensibly for arthritis do not have intrinsic joint disease at all, but rather some form of "nonarticular rheumatism." This imposing designation proves on close scrutiny to be little more than a catch-all category for the assorted aches, pains, and miseries (stiff neck, lumbago, painful shoulder, myalgia, bursitis, and the like) that for generations have provided a bonanza for patent medicine vendors.

Clinicians specializing in arthritis and rheumatology have devised many names to designate certain symptom complexes, with a view to more effective treatment utilizing available potent drugs and numerous physiotherapeutic modalities. This is all right insofar as it goes, provided we do not kid ourselves about it—we know next to nothing about the pathology of so-called fibrositis, myalgia, neuralgia, fasciitis, periarthritis, and so forth. Rheumatologists seem to be in a rut; what they write at present about nonarticular rheumatism is not essentially different than what was said 20 years ago.

It is my impression that, in attempt-

ing broad coverage of problems in differential diagnosis, they have apparently overextended themselves. Conditions such as calcification of tendons (especially the supraspinatus), "frozen" shoulder, Sudeck's atrophy, and infarcts of bone hardly fall within the purview of "rheumatism," while still others, such as fibroplasia of palmar fascia (leading to Dupuytren's contracture), stenosing tenovaginitis, chronic bursitis, joint bodies, neoplasms, pigmented villonodular synovitis, and tenosynovitis, which are also discussed in primers on rheumatic diseases, are perhaps best left to the orthopedist, particularly since the treatment of choice may well be surgery.

Joint manifestations in some hypersensitivity reactions

One can produce a simple hypersensitivity reaction in the rabbit's knee joint as an experimental model by sensitizing the animal to scarlatinal toxin and then, after 10 days, injecting a drop or two of the toxin into the joint. Within a few days the synovial lining shows edema and an eosinophil infiltrate. This reaction disappears within a week if the challenge is not repeated, leaving only slight subsynovial fibrosis as a residuum.

In man, hypersensitivity reactions in joints may occur in susceptible individuals following the administration of *drugs,* such as the sulfonamides and penicillin, as well as in *serum sickness.* Such affected joints may be painful and tender, but the reaction is apparently self-limited. The opportunity to examine tissue specimens in these circumstances seldom presents itself, and the precise nature of the pathologic response appears to be conjectural.

The phenomenon of *intermittent hydrarthrosis* can, in some cases at least, reflect hypersensitivity or allergy to certain foods— shellfish and English walnuts specifically have been implicated as offending allergens. There are well documented cases in which their ingestion precipitated ephemeral knee joint effusion and in which this could be reproduced at will by dietary indiscretion.

As previously noted, rheumatic fever is commonly initiated by an antecedent group A hemolytic streptococcal infection. In some of the other systemic connective tissue diseases with joint manifestations, it would appear that a hypersensitivity factor is operative, although the problem of pathogenesis as a whole is variable and complex.

Chondrocalcinosis (pseudogout)

In chondrocalcinosis, a curious, apparently familial disease described in recent years,[23] there is a tendency for roentgenographically discernible calcium salts to be deposited intermittently in articular cartilage of the knee and other joints, and occasionally elsewhere. In the acute phase, there may be painful swelling of affected joints. As in gout, the attacks may be triggered by a variety of predisposing circumstances. Crystals of calcium combined with phosphate as calcium pyrophosphate dihydrate are found also in the synovial fluid; this apparently is of diagnostic value. The crystals exhibit a positive birefringence with polarized light.[24] The disorder pursues a prolonged course generally through adult life, and its pathogenesis in genetic and biochemical terms is still speculative.

Relapsing polychondritis

In relapsing polychondritis, an unusual recurrent disorder, reports of which are to be found in German and English literature dating back to 1923, there is a remarkable tendency for cartilage structures in many sites to undergo inflammation, dissolution, and, eventually, connective tissue replacement. In articular cartilage, this may lead to clinical arthritis, sometimes deforming and severe. Other untoward sequelae are collapse or distortion of the external ears, the cartilagenous portion of the nose, the laryngeal cartilages, the cartilage rings of the trachea and bronchi (complicated by suffocation and infection), and sometimes the cartilage of the ribs and spinal articulations. That this is more than a papain-like effect is evidenced by the fact that certain noncartilagenous structures, such as the middle ear, the sclera, and the anterior uveal tract, are often involved.

The etiology of this disease remains obscure, although it is noteworthy that corticosteroids are effective in controlling the disease. For a more detailed, informative account, the reader may have recourse to the paper by Pearson and his associates.[25]

Chondromatosis of joints

On occasion, innumerable small foci of hyaline cartilage (and sometimes of bone

Fig. 15-21. Roentgenogram showing synovial chondromatosis (or osteochondromatosis) in an elbow.

as well) may be formed by nodular condensation and metaplasia of the synovial and
subsynovial connective tissue of joints. The
most frequent site for this is the knee joint,
although occasionally a hip, elbow, or some
other joint may be affected. Essentially the
same process may develop in the linings of

bursal sacs or tendon sheaths, but this is
comparatively uncommon.

When a knee joint is involved, for example, one may observe on surgical exploration that the synovium of the joint proper—
and perhaps of the suprapatellar pouch and
posterior compartment as well—is studded

Fig. 15-22. A, Synovial chondromatosis (knee joint). Some of the chondral bodies are
partially calcified, but there was no osseous metaplasia in this particular instance. B,
Another example of synovial chondromatosis. The large, calcified chondral body (on the
left) is ready to pop. The two small bodies have been formed through focal nodular
condensation of the synovial connective tissue, and the larger of the two shows incipient
bone formation in its center.

by small, firm, flat or slightly raised, gray-yellow nodules. These have a tendency to be extruded so that the joint may contain numerous, sometimes hundreds of, free chondral bodies. Whether or not they are visualized roentgenographically depends upon whether they show sufficient calcification or osseous transformation to be radiopaque (Fig. 15-21).

On microscopic examination of the lining of an affected joint, one observes numerous foci of cartilagenous and/or osseous metaplasia in varying stages of development. The cartilage foci, as noted, may become

calcified or converted to bone (Fig. 15-22).

The treatment of choice is synovectomy, as complete as possible, and of course flushing out of all free joint bodies. Malignant change (to chondrosarcoma) has been reported,[26] but it is very unusual.[27]

Pigmented villonodular synovitis

Pigmented villonodular synovitis, which Jaffe, Sutro, and I clarified and christened in 1941,[28] represents essentially a peculiar, self-limited histiocytosis of as yet undetermined etiology, affecting the linings of joints (as well as tendon sheaths and occasionally

Fig. 15-23. Photomicrograph of a field from a lesion of pigmented villonodular synovitis of a knee joint illustrating prominent synovial-lined spaces within the thickened synovial membrane. (Other fields showed appreciable collagenization, scattered multinuclear giant cells, and abundant hemosiderin deposition.)

bursae) in either localized or more diffuse forms. The proliferating stromal cells, which are of dual synovial and adventitial reticular origin, may flourish in tumor-like aggregates early in the cycle of evolution. However, even at this stage, they manifest their phagocytic nature by taking up hemosiderin pigment granules and sometimes lipid. While a variable number of multinuclear (giant) cells may be present, these constitute a minor, secondary feature. Eventually, many lesions tend spontaneously to involute, in part or throughout, and undergo extensive fibrosis and collagenization. This cycle may go on to substantial completion (as it commonly does in tendon sheath nodes of long standing), or it may renew itself, as it does in the more exuberant diffuse lesions in the knee joint. In the process, the synovium and the sublining tissues are more or less deeply pigmented, often becoming deep red-brown

or a chocolate-brown. Collaterally, in the diffuse lesions at least, the affected area is transformed into a tangled, spongy mat or web, often intricately associated with protruding sessile or pedicled nodules (Figs. 15-23 and 15-24).

The condition is not nearly so common in synovial joints as it is in tendon sheaths. The knee joint is most often involved, although occasionally a hip, ankle, or some other joint may be affected. The symptoms are pain, swelling, and sometimes locking of the joint; they may persist for months or even several years before the condition is recognized. Clinically and radiographically there is evidence of a thickened, swollen joint capsule with effusion. The latter tends to recur after tapping and to be serosanguineous; this fact often affords a valuable diagnostic lead. In recent years, it has become increasingly evident that the lesion

Fig. 15-24. Section of a node from a tendon sheath of a finger (pigmented nodular tenosynovitis) showing histiocytic proliferation, occasional syncytial (giant) cells, and focal hemosiderin deposition.

may extend into the contiguous articular bone ends,[29] apparently through eroded apertures in the cortex, in much the same way as tendon sheath nodes of long standing may erode adjacent bones (Fig. 15-25).

In referring to the condition, some commentators drop the qualifying adjective "pigmented," but I find this objectionable since "villonodular synovitis" is too nondescript to constitute a meaningful designation. Also, with reference to dissent, I reject the suggestions that the lesion represents a sclerosing hemangioma, that it represents a benign (giant cell) synovioma in the sense of a genuine neoplasm, or that it results from chronic hemarthrosis. The weight of pathologic evidence is against these views, as has been previously indicated.[28] With reference to the last notion particularly, it may be emphasized that

while repeated hemorrhage into a joint does, to be sure, induce villous hypertrophy and hemosiderin deposition in the lining, it does *not* provoke diffuse histiocytic proliferation. This is as true in experimental models as it is in hemophilia.

Localized lesions of pigmented villonodular synovitis can be readily excised. For diffuse lesions, total synovectomy is the treatment of choice, to be repeated in the event that the condition recurs, as sometimes happens. For these exuberant, recurrent lesions, roentgen therapy affords effective control. As small a tissue dose as 1,500 rads may suffice, but at times a total of 2,000 to 2,500 rads may be necessary. As for malignant change, it is conceivable that this may happen (as it does on rare occasions in old, neglected tendon sheath nodes), but it would be remarkable. I have not observed it to date in my own experience.

Fig. 15-25. Roentgenogram of knee joint region in a case of long-standing pigmented villonodular synovitis. From this picture, one may anticipate finding extension of the lesion into the articular bone ends.

References

1. Sotelo-Ortiz, F.: Chronic coccidioidal synovitis of knee joint, J. Bone Joint Surg. 37-A:48, 1955.
2. Anderson, S. G., Doherty, R. L., and Carley, J. G.: Med. J. Aust. 1:173, 1961.
3. Caranasos, G. J., and Felker, J. R.: Mumps arthritis, Arch. Intern. Med. 119:394, 1967.
4. Filpi, R. G., and Houts, R. L.: Mumps arthritis, J.A.M.A. 205:216, 1968.
5. Chambers, R. J., and Bywaters, E. G. L.: Rubella synovitis, Ann. Rheum. Dis. 22:263, 1963.
6. Committee of the American Rheumatism Association: Primer on the rheumatic diseases: part III, J.A.M.A. 171:1680, 1959.
7. Sokoloff, L., and Bunim, J. J.: Clinical and pathological studies of joint involvement in sarcoidosis, New Eng. J. Med. 260:841, 1959.
8. Case records of the Massachusetts General Hospital, New Eng. J. Med. 263:93, 1960.
9. Collins, D. H.: Haemosiderosis and haemochromatosis of synovial tissues, J. Bone Joint Surg. 33:436, 1951.
10. Roy, S.: Ultrastructure of articular cartilage in experimental hemarthrosis, Arch. Path. 86:69, 1968.
11. Van der Korst, J. K., Sokoloff, L., and Miller, E. J.: Senescent pigmentation of cartilage and degenerative joint disease, Arch. Path. 86:39, 1968.

12. Hollander, J. L., McCarty, D. J., Astorga, G., and Castro-Marillo, E.: Studies on the pathogenesis of rheumatoid joint inflammation: the "R.A. cell" and a working hypothesis, Ann. Intern. Med. **62**:271, 1965.
13. Rawson, A. J., Quismoria, F. P., and Abelson, N. M.: The induction of synovitis in the normal rabbit with Fab: a possible experimental model of rheumatoid arthritis, Amer. J. Path. **54**:95, 1969.
14. Gardner, D. L.: The pathology of polyarthritis. In Symposium; polyarthritis, The Royal College of Physicians of Edinburgh, 1964.
15. Sokoloff, L., McCluskey, R. T., and Bunim, J. J.: Vascularity of the early subcutaneous nodule of rheumatoid arthritis, Arch. Path. **55**:475, 1953.
16. Chandler, G. N., Jones, D. T., Wright, V., and Hartfall, S. J.: Charcot's arthropathy following intra-articular hydrocortisone, Brit. Med. J., p. 952, 1959.
17. Romanus, R.: Pelvo-spondylitis ossificans, Chicago, 1968, Year Book Medical Publishers.
18. Massell, B. F., Honikman, L. H., and Amezcua, J.: Rheumatic fever following streptococcal vaccination, J.A.M.A. **207**:1115, 1969.
19. Rich, A. R., and Gregory, J. E.: Experimental evidence that lesions with basic characteristics of rheumatic carditis can result from anaphylactic hypersensitivity, Bull. Johns Hopk. Hosp. **73**:239-264, 1943.
20. Cruickshank, B.: Ann. Rheum. Dis. **18**:111, 1959.
21. Aegerter, E., and Kirkpatrick, J. A.: Orthopedic diseases, Philadelphia, 1963, W. B. Saunders Co., p. 753.
22. Freyberg, R. H.: Nonarticular rheumatism: the musculoskeletal system: a symposium, New York, 1952, The Macmillan Co., pp. 271-286.
23. McCarty, D. J., Jr., Kohn, N., and Faires, J.: The significance of calcium phosphate crystals in the synovial fluid of arthritic patients: the "pseudogout syndrome," Ann. Intern. Med. **56**:711, 1962.
24. Bluhm, G. B.: Laboratory diagnosis of crystalline arthritis, Bull. Path. Amer. Soc. Clin. Path. **10**:91, 1969.
25. Pearson, C. M., Kline, H. M., and Newcomer, V. D.: Relapsing polychondritis, New Eng. J. Med. **263**:51, 1960.
26. Mullins, F., Berard, C. W., and Eisenberg, J. H.: Chondrosarcoma following synovial chondromatosis, Cancer **18**:1180, 1965.
27. Goldman, R. L., and Lichtenstein, L.: Synovial chondrosarcoma, Cancer **17**:1223, 1964.
28. Jaffe, H. L., Lichtenstein, L., and Sutro, C. J.: Pigmented villonodular synovitis, bursitis and tenosynovitis, Arch. Path. **91**:731, 1941.
29. Breimer, C. W., and Freiberger, R. H.: Bone lesions associated with villonodular synovitis, Amer. J. Roentgen. **79**:618, 1958.

Index*

A

Abscess
  Brodie's, 42
  chronic bone, 38, *40-41*, 42, *45*
  ray fungus and, 53
Achondroplasia, 24-25, *26, 27*
Acidosis, renal disease and, 100
Acromegaly, 73, *74*
  osteoporosis and, 104
Actinomycosis, 50, 52
"Acute atrophy of bone" in posttraumatic rarefaction of bone, 170
Acute disseminated histiocytosis X, 141-143
Acute infectious arthritis, 188-189, *189*
Acute intermittent porphyria, 97
Acute osteomyelitis, 38, 42, *43*
Adenoma
  basophil cell, of anterior lobe of pituitary, 73
  parathyroid, primary hyperparathyroidism and, *80*, 81, 83
Adolescent coxa vara, 161
Adrenal cortical tumors, osteoporosis and, 105
Adrenal glands, 75
Air embolism, bone infarcts and, 165
Albers-Schönberg disease, 20-22, *23*
Albright's syndrome, 14
Albumin, serum, in osteoporosis, 104
Alkaline phosphatase activity; *see* Phosphatase
Alkaptonuria, 94
Allopurinol, 91
Amino acids, renal disease and, 102
Aminoaciduria, 22, 102
Amphotericin B, 192
Amputation neuroma, 159, *159*
Amyloid deposits in infections, 97
Amyloidosis
  atypical, 97
  chronic osteomyelitis and, 44
  rheumatoid arthritis and, 204

Anaplastic tumor, Paget's disease and, 131
Androgen, Paget's disease and, 125
Anemias
  chemical poisoning and, 146
  chronic hemolytic, 117-120, *118, 119, 120*
  familial hemolytic, 120
  hypochromic, Gaucher's disease and, 87
  myelophthisic, and osteopetrosis, 21
  refractory, in vitamin A deficiency, 60
  rickets and, 65
  sickle cell, 117-118
    bone abscess and, 43
    bone infarcts and, 165
  in Still's disease, 204
  in vitamin C deficiency, 62
Aneurysmal bone cyst, 180-183, *181, 182*
Angiomatosis, regional, 171
Ankylosing arthritis, 200
Ankylosing spondylitis, 204
  hereditary ochronosis and, 94, 95-96
  Reiter's syndrome and, 193
Ankylosis
  gout and, 92
  intraarticular fractures and, 186
Anomalies of skeletal development, systematized, 10-37
  achondroplasia in, 24-25, 26, *26, 27*, 27
  cleidocranial dysostosis in, 29, 30, *30*
  dysplasia epiphysealis in, 34
  dysplasia epiphysealis multiplex in, 34
  dysplasia epiphysealis punctata in, 34
  familial metaphyseal dysplasia in, 34
  fibrous dysplasia of bone in, 11-17, *12, 13, 15, 16*
  gargoylism in, 30-33, *31, 32*
  hereditary multiple exostosis in, *16*, 17-19, *17, 18*
  melorheostosis in, 33
  metaphyseal dysostosis in, 34
  monomelic medullary osteosclerosis in, 34, *34*
  Morquio's disease in, 25-29, *27, 28*

---

*Numbers in italics represent pages containing illustrations.

213

Index

Anomalies of skeletal development, systematized—cont'd
  osteogenesis imperfecta in, 22-24, *23, 24, 25*
  osteopetrosis in, 20-22, *22, 23*
  osteopoikilosis in, 28, *28,* 29, *29*
  progressive diaphyseal dysplasia in, 33-34
  skeletal enchondromatosis in, 19-20, *19, 20,* 21
  time of appearance of, 10-11
Antibiotics
  in bone infections, 38, 44, 48, 49, 52
  histiocytosis X and, 142
Anticoagulants, hemophilia and, 115
Antihemophilic factor concentrate, 116
Aplastic anemia, benzol poisoning and, 146
Apposition of periosteal new bone; *see* Periosteal apposition
Aromatic diamidines, 54
Arthralgia, villous nonspecific synovitis and, 186
Arthritic manifestations of metabolic disorders, *194, 195,* 196
Arthritic purpura, 196
Arthritis
  acute infectious, 188-189, *189*
  ankylosing, 200
  atrophic, 200
  degenerative, 196
  gonococcal, 189
  hemorrhagic, 196
  hereditary ochronosis and, 94-95
  hypertrophic, 196
  Marie-Strümpell, 204
  proliferative, 200
  pyogenic, 188-189, *189*
  rheumatoid, 200-205, *201, 202, 203*
    juvenile, 204
    and psoriasis, 204-205
    Reiter's syndrome and, 193
  senescent, 196
  septic, 188-189, *189*
  sickle cell anemia and, 117
  suppurative, 188-189, *189*
  tophaceous, 91
  viral infections and, 54-55
  von Bechterew's, 204
Arthritis deformans, 196
Arthrodesis for skeletal tuberculosis, 48, 190
Articular cartilage, traumatic damage to, 113
Atrophic arthritis, 200
Atrophy
  of bone, acute posttraumatic, 170
  disuse, and osteoporosis, 104, 105
  of muscle, posttraumatic, 170
  Sudeck's, 171
Atypical amyloidosis, 97
Autonomous hyperparathyroidism, 102
Avitaminosis C, 61-64, *62-63*
Azotemia, 100

B
B. proteus, 43
Baker's cyst, 161
Bank bone, 179
Basedow's disease, 76
Basophil cell adenoma of pituitary, 73

Benign giant cell tumors, Paget's disease and, 122
Benzol poisoning, 146
Beryllium, effects of, 148
Besnier-Boeck-Schaumann's disease, 193
Biliary cirrhosis, osteoporosis and, 104
Bilirubin, serum, in thalassemia, 119
Bismuth, 146
Blastomyces dermatitidis, 53
Blastomycosis, 50, 53-54
Bleeding
  of gums in vitamin C deficiency, 62
  in hemophilia, control of, 116
  into joints, 115, *116*
Blood cells, red, defects in, 117-120
Blood clotting factors in hemophilia, 115, 116
Blood diseases, skeletal changes in, 115-121
  hemolytic anemias in, 117-120, *118, 119, 120*
  hemophilia in, 115-117, *116*
Blood supply, loss of, in bone, 164-165, 167, 168
Blount's disease, 163, *163*
Bone abscess, chronic, 38, *40-41,* 42, 45
Bone chips
  aneurysmal bone cyst and, 182
  curettement and packing with, *178,* 179
Bone cortex; *see* Cortex
Bone cyst
  aneurysmal, 180-183, *181, 182*
  epidermoid, 180
  unicameral, 175-180, *176, 177, 178, 179*
Bone disease, disappearing, 171
Bone ends
  articular, in Morquio's disease, 27, 28, *28*
  fractured, excessive resorption of, 5
Bone infarcts; *see* Infarcts in bone
Bone marrow; *see* Marrow, bone
Bony prominences, coccidiomycosis and, 51
Bony union, internal, after fracture, 4
Boplant, 179
Bowing of femora and tibiae in rickets, 65
Brachydactyly in pseudo-hypoparathyroidism, 84
Brittle bones, 22-24, *23, 24, 25*
Brodie's abscess, 42
Brown tumor, 79, 81, *82*
Brucella, 188
Brucella suis, 44
Brucellosis, 43
Bulbous amputation neuroma, 159, *159*
Burnett syndrome, 158
Bursitis, chronic, 152-153, *153*

C
Cachectic states, long-standing terminal, 97
Caffey's disease, 55-57, *55-56*
Caisson disease, *164,* 165, 196
Calcific deposits in vitamin D excess, 70
Calcification
  in bone infarcts, 167
  foci of subcutaneous, in pseudo-hypoparathyroidism, 84
  of osteoid in myositis ossificans, 173
  after radiation on bone, 148, *149*
  of soft parts, 157-158
  soft-tissue, after hemodialysis, 102
  in tendons, *156,* 157

Calcinosis, 90-91
Calcium
  concentration of, at fracture site, 3
  deposits of, in tendons, *156*, 157
  in osteoporosis, 105
  serum level of
    in hypoparathyroidism, 83
    in osteomalacia, 70
    in primary hyperparathyroidism, 77, 78, 80
    renal disease and, 100
    in rickets, 65
    in vitamin D excess, 70
  urinary, in hyperthyroidism, 76
Calcium gout, 90-91
Calcium pyrophosphate dihydrate in synovial fluid, 207
Callus formation after fracture
  fibrocartilaginous, 2
  osseous, 2
  primary, 3-4
Calvarium
  fibrous dysplasia of bone and involvement of, 14
  histiocytosis X and defects of, 143
  inclusion cysts and, 180
  ossification of, in cleidocranial dysostosis, 29, *30*
  in Paget's disease, *126, 130*
Calvé's disease, 140
Capillaries, congested, in posttraumatic rarefaction of bone, 171
Capital femoral epiphysis
  bone infarcts in, sickle cell anemia and, 117
  displacement of, in congenital coxa vara, 162
  slipped, 161-162, *162*
Carbon dioxide–combining power in renal disease, 100
Carcinoma of paranasal sinuses or mastoid, 150; *see also* Malignant change; Tumors
Carcinomatosis, metastatic, osteoporosis and, 105
Caries sicca, 48
Cartilage
  articular, traumatic damage to, 113
  costal, in hereditary ochronosis, *96*
  hyaline, islands of, in fibrous dysplasia of bone, 14, *15*
  metaplastic ossification and, 174
Cartilage cap in hereditary multiple exostosis, 17, 18
Cartilage cell proliferation in achondroplasia, 24
Cartilage cores in osteopetrosis, 21-22, *23*
Cartilage plates, premature closure of, 25, *27*
Cartilaginous exostoses, multiple, 17-19
Catabolic hormones, osteoporosis and, 104
Cat-scratch fever, 55
Celiac disease, 65
Cerebral involvement in histiocytosis X, 135, 137, 139, 143, 144
Charcot neuroarthropathy, 108-113
Charcot's joint, 50, 193
Chemical effects on bone, 146-148, *147, 148*
Cherubism, 132
Chickenpox, 55, 193
Chloramphenicol, 49

Cholesterol deposits
  bone infarcts and, 167
  in xanthoma tuberosum multiplex, 90, *90*
Cholesterol level, serum, in xanthoma tuberosum multiplex, 90
Chondrocalcinosis, 207
Chondrodysplasia, hereditary deforming, 17
Chondrodystrophia fetalis, 24-25, *26, 27*
Chondrodystrophic dwarfism, 24-25, *26, 27*
Chondrodystrophy, nomenclature and, 11
Chondromalacia, 196, *197*
Chondromatosis
  of joints, 207-209, *207, 208*
  of tendon sheaths, 157
Chondroosteodystrophy, Morquio-Brailsford type, 25-29, *27, 28*
Chondrosarcoma
  chondromatosis and, 209
  as effect of radiation, 149
  Paget's disease and, 131
  subungual exostosis and, 175
Chondrosarcomatous change in hereditary multiple exostosis, 18-19, *18*
Christian triad, histiocytosis X and, 143
Christmas disease, 115
Chronic acidosis, renal disease and, 100
Chronic bone abscess, 38, *40-41*, 42, 45
Chronic bursitis, 152-153, *153*
Chronic disseminated histiocytosis X, 143-145
Chronic hemarthrosis, 193, 195-196
Chronic hemolytic anemias, 117-120, *118, 119, 120*
Chronic hemolytic jaundice, 120
Chronic lead poisoning, 146
Chronic nonspecific inflammation of tendons and sheaths, 156-157
Chronic osteomyelitis, 38, *39*, 42, *44*
Chronic synovitis
  syphilis and, 50
  villous nonspecific, 184-186, *185*
Cirrhosis
  biliary, osteoporosis and, 104
  of liver, 102
Clavicles
  cleidocranial dysostosis and defect in, 29
  infantile cortical hyperostosis and, 55, *55-56*
Cleidocranial dysostosis, 29, *30*
Clotting factors, blood, in hemophilia, 115, 116
Clutton's joints, 50, 192
Coagulation deficiency diseases, 115
Coccidioides immitis, 51, 52, *53*
Coccidiomycosis, 50-54, *52, 53*, 190-192, *192*
Colchicine, 91
Collagen deposit in Dupuytren's contracture, 160
Collagen disease, bone infarcts and, 165
Compression fracture, eosinophilic granuloma and, 140
Congenital blood diseases, 115-120
Congenital coxa vara, 162-163, *162*
Congenital defects, renal disease and, 102; *see also* Anomalies of skeletal development, systematized
Congenital lues, 49, 50, *50-51*, 192
Congenital porphyria erythropoietica, 96

Congenital pseudoarthrosis of tibia, 163-164, *163*
Congenital syphilis, 49, 50, *50-51*, 132
Congenital torticollis, 161
Conjunctivitis, Reiter's syndrome and, 193
Connective tissue
  defect in development of, osteogenesis imper-
    fecta and, 22
  degeneration of, in lacerated meniscus, 151
  metaplastic ossification in, 174
  of muscle
    fibromatosis in, Dupuytren's contracture and,
      161
    in myositis ossificans, 173
  myxoid degeneration and cystic softening of
    in ganglion formation, 153
    in meniscal cysts, 151
    in tendons, 158-159, *158*
  systemic diseases of, joint manifestations in,
    205-206
  of tendons, pathology of, 157
  thickening of, in chronic bursitis, 152
Contractures
  Dupuytren's, 159-161, *161*
  Volkmann's, 159, *160*
Cooley's erythroblastic anemia, 118
Copper deficiency, 98
Cornea
  clouding of, in gargoylism, 30-31, 32
  scarring of, in vitamin A deficiency, 60
Cortex
  erosion of, hemophilia and, 116
  fibrous defect of, unicameral bone cyst and, 175
  periosteal ossification and lesion of, 174
  sickle cell anemia and changes in, 118, *118*
  subperiosteal resorption of, hyperparathyroidism
    and, 81
  thinning of
    in congenital pseudoarthrosis of tibia, 163
    and expansion, in unicameral bone cyst, 178
    in Gaucher's disease, 87, *88*
Cortical hyperostosis, infantile, 55-57, *55-56*
  versus vitamin A excess, 60, *61*
Corticoids, 104, *105*
Corticotropin, 91
Cortisone, 104, *105*
Costochondral junctions in rickets, *64, 65*
Cotton-wool calvarium, *130*
Coxa anteverta, 161
Coxa vara
  adolescent, 161
  congenital, 162-163, *162*
  Paget's disease and, 131
Coxitis and osteopetrosis, 21
Cranial nerve injury in vitamin A deficiency, 60
Craniotabes, 65
Creatinine levels, serum, in osteogenesis imper-
  fecta, 22
Cretinism, *76*
Cryptococcosis, 50, 54
Curettement
  for eosinophilic granuloma of bone, 138
  and packing with bone chips
    aneurysmal bone cyst and, 180, 182
    unicameral bone cyst and, *178, 179*

Cushing's syndrome, 73, 75, 104
Cutaneous hyperpigmentation and fibrous dysplasia
  of bone, 14
Cutaneous lesions, histiocytosis X and, 135, 139,
  143; *see also* Skin
Cystic softening, bone infarcts and, 167; *see also*
  Connective tissue, myxoid degeneration and
  cystic softening of
Cystine, renal disease and, 102
Cystine storage disease, 96
Cystinosis, 96
Cysts
  aneurysmal bone, 180-183, *181, 182*
  Baker's, 161
  epidermoid, in bone, 180, *181*
  meniscal or parameniscal, 151, *152*
  parasitic diseases and, 54
  unicameral bone, 175-180, *176, 177, 178, 179*

D

Dactylitis
  sickle cell, 117, *118*
  syphilis and, 50
  tuberculous, *46-47*, 48
Deafness
  gargoylism and, 32
  nerve, syphilis and, 50
  and osteogenesis imperfecta, 22, 24
Debré-de Toni-Fanconi syndrome, 66, *66*, 102
Deficiency
  coagulation, diseases of, 115
  copper, 98
  manganese, 98
  of vitamins, skeletal changes in; *see* Vitamin de-
    ficiencies and excesses, skeletal changes in
  zinc, 98
Degenerative arthritis, 196
Degenerative change in tendons, 158, *158*
Degenerative joint disease, 196
Demineralization of bone, hyperthyroidism and, 76
Density of bone
  in osteopetrosis, 20-22
  in progressive diaphyseal dysplasia, 33-34
Dermatitis, Reiter's syndrome and, 193
Dermatomyositis, joint manifestations of, 205
"Desert rheumatism," 192
Destructive foci in histiocytosis X, 137, 138, 139,
  140, 142, 144
Development, skeletal, anomalies of; *see* Anomalies
  of skeletal development, systematized
Diabetes, renal, 102
Diabetes insipidus, histiocytosis X and, 143, 144, 145
Diabetes mellitus, 77
  neurotrophic changes in, 108, *109*
Diagnosis, differential; *see* Differential diagnosis
Diamidines, aromatic, 54
Diaphyseal aclasis, 17-19
Diaphyseal dysplasia, progressive, 33-34
Diaphyseal sclerosis, hereditary multiple, 33-34
Differential diagnosis
  in bone infarcts, 167
  in coccidiomycosis, 52
  in eosinophilic granuloma of bone, 138, 139-140
  in fibrous dysplasia of bone, 14-16

Differential diagnosis—cont'd
  in Gaucher's and Niemann-Pick diseases, 87
  in infantile cortical hyperostosis, 57
  in leprosy, 49
  in myositis ossificans, 174
  in osteopetrosis, 21
  in osteoporosis, 105
  in posttraumatic rarefaction of bone, 171
  in posttraumatic synovitis, 187
  in skeletal tuberculosis, 48
  in subungual exostosis, 175
Digits, stubby, in dysplasia epiphysealis multiplex, 34
2, 5-Dihydroxyphenylacetic acid, 94
Diplococcus pneumoniae, 188
Disappearing bone disease, 171
Discoid meniscus, 151, *152*
Disk tissue, herniated intervertebral, 154, *155, 156*
Disorders of synovial joints; *see* Synovial joints, disorders of
Displacement of vertebral column, 171; *see also* Vertebral column
Disseminated histiocytosis X; *see* Histiocytosis X
Disseminated lupus erythematosus, 205
Disuse atrophy, osteoporosis and, 104, 105
Donovan bodies, 49
Dorsolumbar kyphosis, gargoylism and, 32
Drainage, surgical, in chronic osteomyelitis, 38
Drugs, hypersensitivity reactions to, 206
Dupuytren's contracture, 159-161, *161*
Dwarfing, osteogenesis imperfecta and, 22, *23, 24*
Dwarfism
  chondrodystrophic, 24-25, *26, 27*
  gargoylism and, 32
  hypothyroidism and, 76
  Lorain type of, 75
  in metaphyseal dysostosis, 34
  primary hypogonadism and, 77
  renal disease and, 102
Dyschondroplasia, nomenclature and, 11
Dysostosis
  cleidocranial, 29, *30*
  metaphyseal, 34
Dysostosis multiplex, 30-33, *31, 32*
Dysplasia
  familial metaphyseal, 34
  fibrous
    of bone, 11-17, *12, 13, 15, 16*
    localized hyperostosis and, 132
    unicameral bone cyst and, 175
  progressive diaphyseal, 33-34
Dysplasia epiphysealis multiplex, 34
Dysplasia epiphysealis punctata, 34
Dystrophia adiposogenitalis, 75

E

Eccentroosteochondrodysplasia, 25-29, *27, 28*
Ecchymoses in vitamin C deficiency, 62
Echinococcosis, 54
Elbow, neuroarthropathy and, 109, *112*
Elements, trace, influence of, on skeleton, 97-98
Emboli, bone infarcts and, 165
Enchondroma, calcified, 167

Enchondromatosis, skeletal, 19-20, *19, 20, 21*
Endochondral ossification
  interference with
    in bismuth poisoning, 146
    in congenital syphilis, 49, *50-51*
  stimulation of, in pituitary gigantism, 73
  in vitamin C deficiency, 63, *63*
Endocrine disorders, skeletal changes in, 73-85
  adrenal glands in, 75
  gonads in, 77
  pancreas in, 77
  parathyroid glands in, 77-84
  pineal gland in, 77
  pituitary gland in, 73-75
  thymus in, 77
  thyroid gland in, 76
Endosteal apposition
  in fluoride osteosclerosis, 147
  sickle cell anemia and, 118
Endosteal surface, unicameral bone cyst and, 178-179
Englemann's disease, 33-34
Enteritis, regional, osteomalacia and, 69
Eosinophilic granuloma; *see* Histiocytosis X
Epidermoid cyst in bone, 180, *181*
Epiphyseal cartilage plates, premature closure of, 25, 27
Epiphyseal osteochondritis of growth centers, 167
Epiphyseal separation
  congenital syphilis and, 49, *50-51*
  in vitamin C deficiency, 63-64
Epiphyses
  capital femoral
    bone infarcts in, sickle cell anemia and, 117
    displacement of, in congenital coxa vara, 162
    slipped, 161-162, *162*
  congenital defect in ossification of, 26, 28
  density and irregularity of, 34
  enlargement of, 65
  infarcts in, 168
  premature fusion of, 119
  slipped, 196
  stippled or speckled, 34
  tibial, 163
Erythrocytes, defects in, 117-120
Erythrocytic destruction, thalassemia and, 119
Erythrodontia, 96
Essential hypercholesterolemia, 89-90
Estrogen, Paget's disease and, 125
Estrogen therapy in osteoporosis, 105, 106
Eunuchism, 77
Eunuchoid states, *74,* 104
Excesses
  molybdenum, 98
  of vitamins, skeletal changes in; *see* Vitamin deficiencies and excesses, skeletal changes in
Exophthalmic goiter, 76
Exophthalmos, histiocytosis X and, 143
Exostoses
  hereditary multiple, *16, 17,* 17-19, *18*
  multiple cartilaginous, 17-19
  subungual, 175

Index

F

Facial palsy
 and osteopetrosis, 21
 in vitamin A deficiency, 60
Facies, grotesque, gargoylism and, 32
Factors, blood, 115, 116
Fallout, radioactive, 150
Familial hemolytic anemia, 120
Familial hyperlipoproteinemia, 90
Familial hyperostosis, 133, *133*
Familial incidence in skeletal anomalies, 10
Familial metaphyseal dysplasia, 34
Fascia, fibromatosis of, Dupuytren's contracture
 and, 159-161, *161*
Felty's syndrome, 204
Femora
 flaring or fusiform expansion of, 87, *88*, 89
 unicameral bone cysts and, *176*, 177
Femoral epiphyses, capital
 bone infarcts in, sickle cell anemia and, 117
 displacement of, in congenital coxa vara, 162
 slipped, 161-162, *162*
Femoral head, bone infarcts in, 165, *166*
Fibrocartilaginous callus, conversion of procallus
 to, 2
Fibroma, nonossifying, unicameral bone cyst and,
 177
Fibromatosis colli, 161
Fibromatosis of palmar and plantar fascia, 159,
 160, 161, *161*
Fibroplasia of palmar and plantar fascia, 159, 160,
 161, *161*
Fibrosarcoma
 chronic osteomyelitis and, 48
 as effect of radiation, 149
 Paget's disease and, 131
Fibrous cortical defect, unicameral bone cyst and,
 175
Fibrous dysplasia of bone, 11-17, *12, 13, 15, 16*
 localized hyperostosis and, 132
 unicameral bone cyst and, 175
Fibrous replacement in chronic osteomyelitis, 38,
 42
Fibrous tissue, Volkmann's contracture and, 159
Fibrous union in congenital pseudoarthrosis, 163
Fingers
 calcinosis of, 157-158, *157*
 inclusion cysts and, 180, *181*
Fluoride, effects of, on bone, 147
Focal nodular histiocytosis, 142, *142*
Foot bones, posttraumatic rarefaction of, 170
Forme fruste
 of fibrous dysplasia, 11, 12
 of hereditary multiple exostosis, 17
Fracture fragment, necrotic, 7
Fracture site
 concentration of calcium and phosphorus at, 3
 organization of hematoma at, 2
 pathologic picture at, 2-3
Fractured bone ends, resorption of, 5
Fractures
 bone infarcts and, 164
 chronic osteomyelitis as complication, 38
 compression, eosinophilic granuloma and, 140

Fractures—cont'd
 congenital pseudoarthrosis of tibia and, 163
 definition of, 1
 fibrous repair in, *1*
 intraarticular, joint changes and, 186
 multiple osteoarticular, 109
 Paget's disease and, 125
 pathologic, 7-9, *8*
 fibrous dysplasia and, 14
 Gaucher's disease and, 87
 hemophilia and, 116
 unicameral bone cyst and, 178, 180
 rickets and, 65
 and sequelae, 1-9
 formation of primary callus in, 3-4
 healing in, 1, 2-4, *2, 3, 4*
 internal bony union in, 4
 nonunion in, 4-7, *6*
 wedge, osteoporosis and, 105
Fragilitas ossium, 22-24, *23, 24, 25*
Fröhlich type of plumpness, 75
Fungus infections, bone involvement in, 50-54, *52,*
 53

G

Ganglion formation, 153-154, *154*
Gargoylism, 29, 30-33, *31, 32*
Garré type of osteomyelitis, *42*
Gas embolism, bone infarcts and, 165
Gastrectomy, osteoporosis and, 104
Gastrointestinal operations, osteomalacia and, 69
Gaucher's disease, 86, 87-89, *88, 89*, 165, 196
"Generalized osteitis fibrosa cystica," 81
Genetic defects, 10; *see also* Anomalies of skeletal
 development, systematized
German measles, 55
Gigantism
 localized, 132
 pituitary, 73, *74*
Glands
 adrenal, 75
 gonads in, 77
 pancreas in, 77
 parathyroid, 77-84
 pineal, 77
 pituitary, 73-75
 thymus in, 77
 thyroid, 76
Glomerulonephritis, 102
Glycine, renal disease and, 102
Glycosuria, 102
Goiter, exophthalmic, 76
Gonadal dysgenesis, osteoporosis and, 104, 105
Gonads, 77
Gonococcal arthritis, 189
Gonococcus, 188
Goundou, 132
Gout, 90-93
 lipid, 89-90, 91
 oxalic, 91
 tophaceous, 91-93
Granulation tissue
 in infantile cortical hyperostosis, *56,* 57
 tuberculous, 190, *190*

Granuloma, eosinophilic; *see* Histiocytosis X
Granuloma inguinale, 49
Graves' disease, 76
Growth zone, broadening of, in vitamin C deficiency, *62-63*, 63
Gummas, 49-50
Gums, bleeding and ulceration of, in vitamin C deficiency, 62

H

Haemophilus influenzae, 188
Hand bones, posttraumatic rarefaction of, 170
Hands, trident, 24, *26*
Healing of fracture, stages of, 1, *2-4, 2, 3, 4*
Hemangiomas, 19, 171
Hemarthrosis
  chronic, joint damage from, 193, 195-196
  in hemophilia, 116
Hematomas
  hemophilia and, 116
  organization of, at fracture site, 2
  ossifying, 174
Hemodialysis, 102
Hemoglobins, abnormal, 117, 118, 119
Hemolytic anemias, 117-120
Hemophilia, 115-117, *116,* 174
Hemorrhages
  hemophilia and, 115-117
  subperiosteal, periosteal ossification and, 174
  in vitamin C deficiency, 62, *62-63,* 63
Hemorrhagic arthritis, 196
Hemosiderosis, joint damage from, 193, 195-196
Hepatomegaly in vitamin A excess, 60
Hepatosplenomegaly
  gargoylism and, 32
  and osteopetrosis, 21
  thalassemia and, 119
Hereditary blood disease, 115-120
Hereditary deforming chondrodysplasia, 17
Hereditary multiple diaphyseal sclerosis, 33-34
Hereditary multiple exostosis, *16,* 17-19, *17, 18*
Hereditary ochronosis, 93-96, *94, 95, 96*
  arthritic manifestations, 195, 196
Hereditary spherocytosis, 119-120
Heredity, 10; *see also* Anomalies of skeletal development, systematized
Herniated intervertebral disk tissue, 154, *155,* 156
Hip joints, neuroarthropathy and, 108, *111*
Hirsutism, 75
Histiocytosis X, 135-145
  acute or subacute disseminated, 141-143
  chronic disseminated, *136,* 143-145, *144*
  classification of, 135
  eosinophilic granuloma of bone in, 137-141, *137, 138, 139, 140, 141, 142, 143, 145*
  etiology of, 136-137
  extraskeletal involvement in, 135-145
Histoplasmosis, 50, 54
Homogentisic acid, 94
Hormones; *see also* Endocrine disorders, skeletal changes in
  catabolic, osteoporosis and, 104
  pituitary growth, 75

Hormones—cont'd
  sex, diminution or loss of, 104, 105
Humerus, unicameral bone cyst and, *176,* 177, *177, 178, 179*
Hunger osteopathy, 67
Hurler-Pfaundler disease, 30-33, *31, 32*
Hurler's syndrome, 30-33, *31, 32*
Hutchinson's teeth, 50
Hyaline cartilage
  cap of, in hereditary multiple exostosis, 17, 18
  islands of, in fibrous dysplasia of bone, 14, *15*
  tumors of, in skeletal enchondromatosis, 19
Hyalinization after radiation, 148
Hydrarthrosis, intermittent, 206
Hydrocephalus, 60
Hydronephrosis, 102
25-Hydroxycholecalciferol, 70
Hypercalcemia, 70, 77
Hypercalcuria
  osteoporosis and, 105
  Paget's disease and, 125
Hypercholesterolemia, essential, 89-90
Hypercorticism, 75
Hyperlipoproteinemia, familial, 90
Hyperostoses
  acquired syphilis and, 50, *50-51*
  affecting skull particularly, 132-133
  familial, 133, *133*
  infantile cortical, 55-57, *55-56,* 60, *61*
  in melorheostosis, 33
Hyperostosis corticalis generalisata, 133
Hyperostosis frontalis interna, 132
Hyperoxaluria, primary, 96
Hyperparathyroidism
  autonomous, 102
  primary, 77-83, *78, 79, 80, 82*
  secondary, 83, 100, 102
  tertiary, 102
  unicameral bone cyst and, 177
Hyperphosphaturia, osteomalacia and, 69
Hyperpigmentation and fibrous dysplasia of bone, 14
Hyperplastic bone marrow, 117, 119
Hypersensitivity reactions, joint manifestations of, 206-207
Hyperthyroidism, 76
Hypertrophic arthritis, 196
Hypertrophic osteoarthropathy, 175
Hyperuricemia in gout, 91
Hypervitaminosis A, 60-61, *61*
Hypervitaminosis D, 70
Hypochromic anemia, Gaucher's disease and, 87
Hypogenesis, 102
Hypogonadal osteoporosis, 104, 105
Hypogonadism, primary, 77
Hypo-hyperparathyroidism, 84
Hypoparathyroidism, 83-84
Hypophosphatasia, 67
Hypophosphatemic–vitamin D refractory rickets, 66, *66,* 102
Hypophyseal infantilism, 75
Hypophyseal involvement, histiocytosis X and, 135, 143, 144

Index

Hypopituitarism, 75
Hypothyroidism, 76

I

Icterus, chronic hemolytic anemias and, 119, 120
Idiopathic osteoporosis, 104
Idiopathic steatorrhea, 65
Iliac crest, bone chips from, 179
Immobilization, disuse atrophy from, 104
Inclusion cysts, 180
Industrial hazards, 146-148
Infantile cortical hyperostosis, 55-57, 55-56, 60, 61
Infantile vitamin D–deficiency rickets, 100, 101
Infantilism, renal disease and, 102
Infarcts in bone, 164-167, 164, 165, 166
  in juvenile osteochondritis, 167, 168, 168
  reconstruction of, 167
  sickle cell anemia and, 117, 118
Infections
  bacterial, secondary to histiocytosis X, 142-143
  of bone, 38-59
    fungus infections in, 50-54, 52, 53
    granuloma inguinale in, 49
    infantile cortical hyperostosis in, 55-57, 55-56, 60, 61
    leprosy in, 48-49, 108, 110
    parasitic disease in, 54
    pathologic reaction to, 38, 42
    pyogenic osteomyelitis in, 38-48, 39, 40, 41, 42, 43, 44, 45
    syphilis in, 49-50, 50, 51, 108-109, 132
    tuberculosis in, 46, 47, 48
    viral infections in, 54-55
  in etiology of histiocytosis X, 136-137
  of joints, 188-193, 189, 190, 191, 192
  long-standing, metabolic disorders and, 97
  in nonunion of fractures, 5
Inflammation
  of joints, 188-189
  rheumatoid, 157
  of tendons and sheaths, 156-157
Inflammatory osteoperiostitis, infantile cortical hyperostosis and, 55-57, 55-56
Infractions, Paget's disease and, 125, 131
Injury
  joint changes following, 186-188, 186, 187
  to knee and lacerated meniscus, 151
  periosteal ossification and, 174
Innominate bone, eosinophilic granuloma and, 140
Intermittent hydrarthrosis and hypersensitivity reactions, 206
Internal bony union after fracture, 4
Interstitial keratitis, syphilis and, 50
Intervertebral disk tissue, herniated, 154, 155, 156
Intestinal malabsorption in osteomalacia, 69
Intraarticular fractures, 186
Intramedullary hemorrhage, 116
Iproniazid, 48
Iron, serum, in thalassemia, 119
Irradiation; see also Roentgen therapy
  in chronic disseminated histiocytosis X, 145
  effects of, on bone, 148-150
  roentgen, aneurysmal bone cyst and, 182

J

Jaundice
  hemolytic anemias and, 119, 120
  histiocytosis X and, 144
Joint bodies
  formation of, 187-188, 187
  after fractures, 7
Joint capsules
  ganglion formation in, 153, 154
  metaplastic ossification and, 174
"Joint mice," 188, 196
Joints; see also Synovial joints, disorders of
  acromegaly and changes in, 73-74
  bleeding into, 115, 116
  Charcot, 50, 193
  chondromatosis of, 207-209, 207, 208
  chronic hemarthrosis and damage to, 193, 195-196
  Clutton's, 192
  coccidiomycosis of, 190-192, 192
  degenerative disease of, 196
  destruction of, 108-113
  gout and, 91-93
  hemorrhages about, in vitamin C deficiency, 62
  in hypersensitivity reactions, 206-207
  infections of, 188-193, 189, 190, 191, 192
  knee
    in avascular necrosis of bone, 168
    Baker's cyst and, 161
    fungus infection and, 54
  lumbosacral, spondylolisthesis and, 171
  neurotrophic disorders of, 196
  sarcoidosis and, 193
  syphilis and, 50, 192-193
  in systemic connective diseases, 205-206
  trauma and changes in, 186-188, 186, 187
  tuberculosis of, 189-190, 190, 191
  in viral diseases, 193
"Juvenile osteochondritis," avascular necrosis in, 167-170, 167, 168, 169
Juvenile Paget's disease, 124
Juvenile rheumatoid arthritis, 204
Juvenile taboparesis, 50

K

Kerasin, 87
Keratitis
  interstitial, syphilis and, 50
  in vitamin A deficiency, 60
Klebsiella pneumoniae, 43
Knee joints
  in avascular necrosis in "juvenile osteochondritis," 168
  Baker's cyst and, 161
  bleeding into, 115-116, 116
  chronic synovitis and, 50
  fungus infection and, 54
  menisci of, pathology of, 151, 152
  neuroarthropathy and, 108, 111, 112
Kümmell's disease, 171
Kyphoscoliosis, Paget's disease and, 131
Kyphosis
  acromegaly and, 73, 74
  gargoylism and, 32

Kyphosis—cont'd
  in Morquio's disease, 28
  osteoporosis and, 105
  Paget's disease and, *124*
  sickle cell anemia and, 118

L

Lacerated menisci, 151, *152,* 196
Lantern jaw, 73
Late rickets, 66
Lead poisoning, 146, *147*
Leg ulcers, sickle cell anemia and, 117
Legg-Perthes' disease, 168, *168*
Leontiasis ossea, 132-133
Leprosy
  neurotrophic changes in, 108, *110*
  skeletal changes in, 48-49
Léri type of osteopetrosis, 33
Letterer-Siwe disease; *see* Histiocytosis X
Leukemia
  effects of radiation and, 148, 150
  histiocytosis X and, 142
Leukocytes in eosinophilic granuloma, 140, *140*
Leukoderma, syphilis and, 50
Leukopenia, Gaucher's disease and, 87
Lignac-Fanconi disease, 96
Limb bones; *see* Long limb bones
Lipid in bone, infarcts and, 165
Lipid gout, 89-90, 91
Lipid metabolism, primary disorders of, 86-90
Lipochondrodystrophy, 30-33, *31, 32*
Lipoglycoprotein storage disease, 31
"Lipogranulomatosis," 97
Liver
  cirrhosis of, 102
  histiocytosis X and, 136, *136,* 144
Lobstein's syndrome, 22-24, *23, 24, 25*
Localized gigantism, 132
Locomotor ataxia, 108
Long limb bones
  aneurysmal bone cyst and, 180, *181*
  enlargement of ends of, 34
  eosinophilic granuloma of bone and, *137, 138,* 140
  in familial metaphyseal dysplasia, 34
  fractures of, in rickets, 65
  infantile cortical hyperostosis and, 55, *55-56*
  infarcts and, 164, 165, 166, 167
  lead poisoning and, 146
  metaphyses of, rubella and, 55
  posttraumatic rarefaction of bone and, 171
  in progressive diaphyseal dysplasia, 33
  sclerosis and widening of, 33
  spherocytic anemia and, 120
  thalassemia and, 119, *120*
  transverse line on growth plates of, 146, *147*
  unicameral bone cysts and, *176,* 177, *177, 178, 179*
Looser zones in osteomalacia, *68, 69*
Lorain type of dwarfism, 75
Lues, congenital, 49, 50, *50-51*
Lumbar spine, pain in, osteoporosis and, 104
Lumbosacral joint, spondylolisthesis and, 171

Lung, histiocytosis X and, 135, 136, 142-143, 144, 145
Lupus erythematosus, joint manifestations of, 205
Lymph nodes
  in eosinophilic granuloma, 142, *142*
  histiocytosis X and, 144
Lymphadenopathy
  in rickets, 65
  and Still's disease, 204
Lymphoid tissue, eosinophilic granuloma and, *141*

M

Macrogenitosomia praecox, 77
Madura foot, 48
Maffucci's syndrome, 19
Malignant change
  chondromatosis and, 209
  in fibrous dysplasia of bone, 16, 17
  in hereditary multiple exostosis, 18-19, *18*
  in old sinus tracts, 44
  in Paget's disease, 131-132
  in pigmented villonodular synovitis, 211
Malignant tumors, osteomyelitis and, 44; *see also* Tumors
Malnutrition, osteoporosis and, 104, 105
Malum coxae senilis, 197
Mandible, infantile cortical hyperostosis and, 55, *55-56*
Manganese, deficiency of, 98
Marble bone disease, 20-22, *23*
Marie-Strümpell arthritis, 204
Marrow, bone
  calcification and necrotic detritus in, 167
  hemorrhages in, in vitamin C deficiency, *62-63,* 63
  hyperplastic, 117, 119
Masculinizing effect in tumors of adrenal gland, 75
Massive osteolysis, 171
Mastoid, carcinoma of, 150
Maxilla, fibrous dysplasia of bone and, 15, 16
Measles, German, 55
Mediterranean anemia, 118
Medullary osteosclerosis, monomelic, 34, *34*
Melorheostosis, 33
"Meningeom-hyperostose," 132
Meningioma en plaque, 132
Meningiomas, localized hyperostosis and, 132
Meningococcus, 188
Meniscal or parameniscal cysts, 151, *152*
Menisci of knee
  pathology of, 151, *152*
  torn, osteoarthritis and, 196
Menopause, osteoporosis and, 104, 105
Mental deficiency
  gargoylism and, 32
  in vitamin A deficiency, 60
Mercury poisoning, 147-148
Mesothorium, bone sarcoma and, 149, 150
Metabolic disorders
  arthritic manifestations of, *194, 195,* 196
  skeletal changes in, 86-99
    gout in, 90-93
    hereditary ochronosis in, 93-96
    porphyria in, 96-97

Metabolic disorders—cont'd
  skeletal changes in—cont'd
    primary disorders of lipid metabolism in, 86-90
    systemic disorders of mucopolysaccharide metabolism in, 97
Metabolic rickets, renal disease and, 102
Metabolism
  disorders of; *see* Metabolic disorders, skeletal changes in
  of mucopolysaccharides
    gargoylism and, 31
    Morquio's disease and, 29
Metaphyseal dysplasia, familial, 34
Metaphyseal dysostosis, 34
Metaphyses
  contiguous, Blount's disease and, 163
  of humerus, unicameral bone cyst and, *176,* 177
  of long bones, rubella and, 55
Metaplastic ossification, 173, 174-175, *174*
Metastatic carcinomatosis, osteoporosis and, 105
Microcrystalline synovitis, 91
Micromelia, 24-25, *26, 27,* 32
Milk-alkali syndrome, 158
Milkman's syndrome, *68,* 69, *69*
Milled bone, 179
Möller-Barlow's disease, 61-64, *62-63*
Molybdenum excess, 98
Monomelic medullary osteosclerosis, 34, *34*
Monostotic fibrous dysplasia, 11, 12, *12*
Monostotic Paget involvement, *123, 127,* 131
Morquio's disease, 25-29, *27, 28*
Morquio-Ullrich disease, 29
"Mosaic" pattern of bone in Paget's disease, 122, 128, *128*
Mottled bone rarefaction, 171
Mottling of teeth, fluoride and, 147
Mucopolysaccharide metabolism
  gargoylism and, 31
  Morquio's disease and, 29
  systemic disorders of, 97
Multiple cartilaginous exostoses, 17-19
Multiple diaphyseal sclerosis, hereditary, 33-34
Multiple exostosis, hereditary, *16,* 17-19, *17*
Multiple myeloma, osteoporosis and, 105
Multiple osteoarticular fractures, 109
Multiple sclerosis, neurotrophic changes in, 108, *109*
Mumps parotitis, 193
Muscle atrophy in posttraumatic rarefaction of bone, 170
Muscle necrosis, Volkmann's contracture and, 159
Muscles, myositis ossificans and, 173
Mycelia in actinomycosis, 53
Mycobacterium leprae, 48
Mycobacterium tuberculosis, 48
Mycotic osteomyelitis, 52-54
Myeloma, multiple, osteoporosis and, 105
Myelophthisic anemia and osteopetrosis, 21
Myositis ossificans, 172-174, *172, 173*
Myxedema, 76
Myxoid degeneration and cystic softening of connective tissue
  in ganglion formation, 153, *154*

Myxoid degeneration and cystic softening of connective tissue—cont'd
  in meniscal cysts, 151
  in tendons, *158,* 158-159

N

Nail bed, subungual exostosis and, 175
Nanosomia pituitaria, 75
Necrobiosis after radiation, 148
Necrosis
  of bone
    bone infarcts and, 164-165, *166,* 167
    after fractures, 5, 7
    in Gaucher's disease, *89*
    in "juvenile osteochondritis," 167-170, *167, 168, 169*
  of muscle, Volkmann's contracture and, 159
  after radiation, 148, 150
Necrotic detritus in marrow, *166, 167, 168*
Necrotic fracture fragment, 7
Neoplastic reticulosis, histiocytosis X and, 142
Nephrocalcinosis, 70, 77, 100
Nephrolithiasis, osteoporosis and, 105
Nerves
  cranial, seventh, in vitamin A deficiency, 60
  peripheral, amputation neuroma and, 159
Neuritis, leprosy and, 48
Neuroarthropathy, 108-113
Neuroma, amputation, 159, *159*
Neurotrophic disorders
  of joints, 196
  skeletal changes in, 108, 114, *109, 110, 111, 112, 113*
New bone
  apposition of, periosteal; *see* Periosteal apposition
  spicules of, sickle cell anemia and, 118
Nicotinic acid hydrazides, 48
Niemann-Pick disease, 86, 87
Nitrogen mustard, histiocytosis X and, 142
Nocardia, 48
Node, Schmorl's, *155,* 156
Nodule, rheumatoid, 203, *203*
Nonarticular "rheumatism," 206
Nonossifying fibroma, 177
Nonsuppurative osteomyelitis, 54
Nonunion after fractures, 4-7, *6*
  inadequate immobilization in, 5
  infection in, 5
  necrotic fragments in, 7, *7*
  pathologic specimens in, 5-7
Nose, saddle, 50

O

Ochronosis, hereditary, 93-96, *94, 95, 96*
Ochronotic ankylosing spondylitis, 95-96
Ollier's disease, 19-20, *19, 20, 21*
Optic atrophy and osteopetrosis, 21
Osgood-Schlatter's disease, 170, *170*
Osseous callus after fractures, 2
Ossification
  endochondral
    in bismuth poisoning, 146
    in congenital syphilis, 49, *50-51*

Ossification—cont'd
  endochondral—cont'd
    in pituitary gigantism, 73
    in vitamin C deficiency, 63, *63*
  metaplastic, 173
  in myositis ossificans, 173-174
  periosteal, 174-175, *174*
Ossifying hematomas, 174
"Osteitis," radiation necrosis and, 150
Osteitis deformans, 122-132; *see also* Paget's disease of bone
Osteitis fibrosa cystica, generalized, 81
Osteoarthritis
  secondary
    hemophilia and, 116, *116*
    hereditary ochronosis and, 95
    neuroarthropathy and, 113
    spondylolisthesis and, 171
    synovial joints and, 196-200, *197, 198, 199*
Osteoarthropathy, hypertrophic, 175
Osteoarthrosis, 196
Osteoarticular destruction, hemophilia and, 116
Osteoarticular fractures, multiple, 109
Osteocartilaginous exostoses, 17-18, *18*
Osteochondritis
  of growth centers, epiphyseal, 167
  syphilis and, 49, *50-51*, 192
Osteochondritis deformans juvenilis, 167
Osteochondritis dissecans, *167*, 168, *168, 169*
  joint bodies and, 188
  osteoarthritis and, 196
Osteochondrodystrophia deformans, 25-29, *27, 28*
Osteochondromas in hereditary multiple exostosis, 17-18, *18*
Osteochondromatosis, 207-209, *207, 208*
  osteoarthritis and, 196
  of synovium, joint bodies and, 188
Osteochondrosis, 167
Osteodystrophy, renal, 66-67, *67*
Osteogenesis imperfecta, 22-24, *23, 24, 25*
Osteogenesis imperfecta fetalis, 22
Osteogenesis imperfecta tarda, 22, 24
Osteogenic sarcoma
  beryllium and, 148
  in complication of Paget's disease, 124, 131
  as effect of radiation, 149, 150
  periosteal ossification and, *174*, 175
Osteoid
  in myositis ossificans, 173, 174
  in osteomalacia, 67, 70
  in rickets, 64, 65, 66
Osteolysis, massive, 171
Osteomalacia, 67-70, *68, 69*
Osteomata, 132
Osteomyelitis
  acute, 38, 42, *43*
  chronic, 38, *39*, 42, *44*
  after fractures, 5
  Garré type of, *42*
  leprous, 49
  mycotic, unusual expressions of, 52-54
  nonsuppurative, viral infections and, 54
  and osteopetrosis, 21
  pyogenic, 38-48, *39, 40, 41, 42, 43, 44, 45*

Osteomyelitis—cont'd
  radiation necrosis and, 150
  in sickle cell anemia, *Salmonella* and, 117, *118*
"Osteomyelitis variolosa," 54
Osteopathia condensans disseminata, *28*, 29
Osteopathia hyperostotica (sclerotisans) multiplex infantilis, 33-34
Osteopenia, 104-107; *see also* Osteoporosis
Osteoperiostitis
  infantile cortical hyperostosis and, 55-57, *55-56*
  syphilis and, 49
Osteopetrosis, 20-22, *22, 23*
  Léri type of, 33
Osteopoikilosis, *28*, 29
Osteoporosis, 104-107, *105, 106*
  Cushing's syndrome and, 73
  hyperthyroidism and, 76
  primary hypogonadism and, 77
Osteoporosis circumscripta cranii, Paget's disease and, 126, *126*
Osteopsathyrosis, 22-24, *23, 24, 25*
Osteosarcoma, subungual exostosis and, 175
Osteosclerosis
  beryllium and, 148
  fluoride and, 147, *148*
  monomelic medullary, 34, *34*
  sickle cell anemia and, 118
Osteosclerosis fragilis, 20-22, *23*
Osteosi eburnizzante monomelica, 33
Otosclerosis, osteogenesis imperfecta and, 24
Ovarian agenesis, 77
Oxalic gout, 91
Oxalism, 91, 96
Oxycephaly
  sickle cell anemia and, 118
  spherocytic anemia and, 120

P

Paget's disease of bone, 122-132, *123, 124, 125, 126, 127, 128, 129, 130, 131*
  clinical considerations in, 122-126
  localized hyperostosis and, 132
  malignant change in, 131-132, *131*
  orthopedic problems in, 125
  pathologic changes in, 126-131
Pain
  acute, sickle cell anemia and, 117
  back, spondylolisthesis and, 172
  in lumbar spine, osteoporosis and, 104
  in melorheostosis, 33
  Paget's disease and, 125
  in posttraumatic rarefaction of bone, 170
  and swelling, myositis ossificans and, 173
Palmar fascia, fibroplasia of, 159, 160, 161, *161*
Palsy, facial, 21, 60
Pancreas, 77
Pancreatitis, osteomalacia and, 69
Parameniscal cysts, 151, *152*
Paranasal sinuses, carcinoma of, 150
Paraplegia, neurotrophic changes in, 108
Parasitic disease, lesions of bone and, 54
Parathyroid adenoma, hyperparathyroidism and, *80*, 81, 83
Parathyroid glands, 77-84

Parotitis, mumps, 193
Parrot's pseudoparalysis, 192
Pathologic fracture; *see* Fractures, pathologic
Pathology
    of bone infections, 38
    and classification of nonarticular "rheumatism,"
       206
    in Paget's disease, 126-131
    of vitamin C deficiency, *62-63, 63*
Pelvospondylitis ossificans, 204
Penicillin, 49, 188
    hypersensitivity reactions to, 206
Periarteritis nodosa, joint manifestations of, 206
Perineuritis, leprosy and, 48
Periosteal apposition
    in fluoride osteosclerosis, 147
    new bone
       in infantile cortical hyperostosis, *55-56, 57*
       metaplastic ossification and, 174-175
       in vitamin A excess, 60, *61*
Periosteal ossification, 174-175, *174*
Periosteal surface, unicameral bone cyst and, 178
Periosteum, hemorrhage in or under
    hemophilia and, 116
    vitamin C deficiency and, *62-63, 63*
Periostitis, syphilis and, 49
Peripheral nerves
    amputation neuroma and, 159
    injury to, 108
Perthes' disease, 167, 196
Phalanges, finger, inclusion cysts and, 180, *181*
Phantom bones, 171
Phenylbutazone, 91
Phosphatase
    activity of
       in hypophosphatasia, 67
       increase in, after fracture, 3
       in osteomalacia, 70
       in rickets, 65
    serum level of
       in Gaucher's disease, 87
       Paget's disease and, 124
       primary hyperparathyroidism and, 81
Phosphate
    and calcium in synovial fluid, 207
    loss of, renal disease and, 102
    retention of, renal disease and, 100
Phosphorus
    concentration of, at fracture site, 3
    effects of, on bone, 146-147
    serum level of
       in hypoparathyroidism, 83
       in osteomalacia, 70
       in rickets, 65
    urinary, in hyperthyroidism, 76
Pigmented villonodular synovitis, 195, 209-211,
    209, 210, 211
Pineal gland, 77
Pinealomas of pineal gland, 77
Pituitary, histiocytosis X and, 135, 143, 144
Pituitary basophilism, 73
Pituitary gigantism, 73, *74*
Pituitary gland, 73-75
Pituitary growth hormone, 75

Plantar fascia, fibroplasia of, 160, 161
Plasma thromboplastin antecedent (PTA), 115
Plasma thromboplastin component (PTC), 115
Platelet cofactor (AHF), 115
Plumbism, 146
Plutonium, bone sarcoma and, 149
Pneumonia in vitamin C deficiency, 62
Podagra, 91
Poisoning
    chemical, 146-148
    vitamin; *see* Vitamin deficiencies and excesses,
       skeletal changes in
Polyarteritis, joint manifestations of, 206
Polyarthritis in children, 204
Polychondritis, relapsing, 207
Polyostotic fibrous dysplasia, 11, 13, *13, 14*
Popliteal space, Baker's cyst and, 161
Porphyria, 96-97
Porphyria cutanea tarda, 97
Porphyria erythropoietica, congenital, 96
Porphyria hepatica, 97
Porphyrins, 96
Postirradiation sarcoma, 149
Postmenopausal osteoporosis, 104, 105
Posttraumatic rarefaction of bone, 170-171
Posttraumatic synovitis, differential diagnosis in,
    187
Pott's disease with gibbus, 48
Pregnancy, osteoporosis and, 104
Primary callus, formation of, 3-4
Primary disorders of lipid metabolism, 86-90
Primary hyperoxaluria, 96
Primary hyperparathyroidism, 77-83
Primary hypogonadism, 77
Probenecid, 91
Procallus, conversion of, to fibrocartilaginous cal-
    lus, 2
Prognathism, acromegaly and, 73, *74*
Progressive diaphyseal dysplasia, 33-34
Proliferative arthritis, 200
Proptosis, Paget's disease and, 125
Proteins, serum, primary hyperparathyroidism and,
    77
Pruriginous rash in vitamin A excess, 60
Pseudoarthrosis, 7
    of tibia, congenital, 163-164, *163*
Pseudofractures, osteomalacia and, *68,* 69, *69*
Pseudogout, 207
Pseudo-hypoparathyroidism, 84
Pseudoparalysis, Parrot's, 192
Pseudo-pseudo-hypoparathyroidism, 84
Psoriasis, rheumatoid arthritis and, 204-205
Pubertas praecox and fibrous dysplasia of bone, 14
Pulmonary lesions, histiocytosis X and, 135, 136,
    142-143, 144, 145
Purpura
    arthritis, 196
    joint damage and, 196
Pyarthrosis, 54, 188-189, *189*
Pyogenic arthritis, 188-189, *189*
Pyogenic osteomyelitis, 38-48, *39, 40, 41, 42, 43,*
    44, 45

R

Radiation effects on bone, 148-150, *149*
Radioactive elements, bone sarcoma and, 149
Radioactive fallout, long-term effects of, 150
Radium, bone sarcoma and, 149, 150
Rarefaction of bone, posttraumatic, 170-171
Rash, pruriginous, in vitamin A excess, 60
Ray fungus, 52-53
Raynaud's phenomenon, 205
Red blood cells, defects in, 117-120
Regional angiomatosis, 171
Regional enteritis, osteomalacia and, 69
Reiter's syndrome, 193
Relapsing polychondritis, 207
Renal diabetes, 102
Renal disease, skeletal changes in, 100-103
Renal osteodystrophy, 66-67, *67*, 100, *101*, 102
Renal osteomalacia, 102
Renal osteosclerosis, 100
Renal rickets, 66-67, *67*
Resorption
    of fractured bone ends, 5
    in Paget's disease, 122
Resorptive skeletal changes, 100, *101*
Retardation, mental and physical, in vitamin A
        deficiency, 60; *see also* Anomalies of skele-
        tal development, systematized
Reticuloendotheliosis, histiocytosis X and, 142
Rheumatic fever, joint manifestations in, 205
"Rheumatism"
    desert, 192
    nonarticular, classification and pathology of, 206
Rheumatoid arthritis, 200-205, *201, 202, 203*
    juvenile, 204
    with psoriasis, 204-205
    Reiter's syndrome and, 193
Rheumatoid inflammation, 157
Rheumatoid nodule, 203, *203*
"Rheumatoid" spondylitis, 204
Ribs, infantile cortical hyperostosis and, 55
Rickets, 64-67, *64, 66, 67*
    hypophosphatasia and, 67
    hypophosphatemic vitamin D–resistant, 102
    infantile vitamin D–deficiency, 100, *101*
    late, *66*
    metabolic, 102
    osteomalacia and, 67-70, *68, 69*
    renal, 66-67, *67*
    renal disease and, 100, *101*, 102
    vitamin D–resistant, 66, *66*, 102
Rickets tarda, 66
Roentgen rays, effects of, on bone, 148-150
Roentgen therapy
    aneurysmal bone cyst and, 182
    for eosinophilic granuloma of bone, 138
    in histiocytosis X, 145
    pigmented villonodular synovitis and, 211
Rubella, 55, 193
Rupture of tendons, traumatic, 158-159, *158*

S

Salmonella infections, 42, *45*, 117, *118*
Sarcoid, tendons and sheaths and, 157
Sarcoidosis, joint involvement and, 193

Sarcoma
    chondromatosis and, 209
    as effect of radiation, 149, 150
    osteogenic
        beryllium and, 148
        in complication of Paget's disease, 124, 131,
            131
        periosteal ossification and, *174, 175*
        Paget's disease and, 122, 124, 131, *131*
        subungual exostosis and, 175
Sarcomatous change in fibrous dysplasia of bone,
        16, 17
Saturnism, 146
Scapulae, infantile cortical hyperostosis and, 55
Scar tissue
    Dupuytren's contracture and, 161
    after radiation, 148
Schmorl's node, *155, 156*
Schüller-Christian disease; *see* Histiocytosis X
Sclera, osteogenesis imperfecta and, 22
Sclerodactyly, 205
Scleroderma, 158, 205-206
Sclerosis
    hereditary multiple diaphyseal, 33-34
    osteogenesis imperfecta and, 22, 24
    in rickets, 65
    sickle cell anemia and, 118
    and widening of long bones in progressive di-
        aphyseal dysplasia, 33
Scorbutus, 61-64, *62-63*
Scurvy, 61-64, *62-63*
    hemarthrosis and, 195
    osteoporosis and, 104
    periosteal ossification and, 174
Secondary hyperparathyroidism, 83
    renal disease and, 100, 102
Secondary hypertrophic arthritis, 196
Secondary osteoarthritis
    gout, and 92
    hemophilia and, 116, *116*
    hereditary ochronosis and, 95
    neuroarthropathy and, 113
Senescent arthritis, 196
Senility, osteoporosis and, 104
Septic arthritis, 188-189, *189*
Sequelae to fractures, 1-9; *see also* Fractures and
        sequelae
Serum albumin in osteoporosis, 104
Serum bilirubin in thalassemia, 119
Serum calcium; *see* Calcium, serum level of
Serum cholesterol in xanthoma tuberosum multi-
        plex, 90
Serum iron in thalassemia, 119
Serum phosphatase; *see* Phosphatase
Serum phosphorus; *see* Phosphorus, serum level of
Serum protein electrophoretic separation, 77
Serum sickness, 206
Sex hormones, osteoporosis and, 104, 105
Shin, saber, 50, 118
Sickle cell anemia, 117-118
    bone abscess and, 43
    bone infarcts and, 165
Sickle cell dactylitis, 117, *118*
Sicklemia, 117

Simmond's disease, 75
Skeletal changes
  in blood diseases, 115-121
    chronic hemolytic anemias in, 117-120
    hemophilia and, 115-117
  in endocrine disorders; *see* Endocrine disorders,
    skeletal changes in
  in granuloma inguinale, 49
  in leprosy, 48-49
  in metabolic disorders; *see* Metabolic disorders,
    skeletal changes in
  in neurotrophic disorders, 108-114
  in renal disease, 100-103
  resorptive, 100, *101*
  in syphilis; *see* Syphilis
  in vitamin deficiencies and excesses; *see* Vitamin
    deficiencies and excesses, skeletal changes
    in
Skeletal development, systematized anomalies of;
  see Anomalies of skeletal development,
  systematized
Skeletal enchondromatosis, 19-20, *19, 20, 21*
Skeletal tuberculosis, *46-47,* 48
Skeleton, influence of trace elements on, 97-98
Skin
  hemangiomas of, and skeletal enchondromatosis,
    19
  histiocytosis X and, 135, 139, 143
  osteogenesis imperfecta and, 22
  radiation and effects on, 148
Skull
  changes in
    acromegaly and, 73-74
    sickle cell anemia and, 118
    spherocytic anemia and, 120
    thalassemia and, 119, *119*
  eosinophilic granuloma of bone and, *139,* 140,
    141
  hyperostoses affecting, 132-133
  Paget's disease and, *126, 130*
  thickening of, in progressive diaphyseal dyspla-
    sia, 33
Slipped epiphysis
  capital femoral, 161-162, *162*
  osteoarthritis and, 196
Slipping vertebra, 171
Smallpox, 54
Spherocytic anemia, 119-120
Spherocytosis, hereditary, 119-120
Spicules of new bone, sickle cell anemia and, 118
Spina bifida, neurotrophic changes in, 108
Spina ventosa, *46-47,* 48
Spinal cord, syrinx of, neuroarthropathy and, 113
Spinal cord damage, neurotrophic changes in, 108,
  110
Spine; *see also* Vertebrae; Vertebral bodies; Ver-
    tebral column
  Charcot, 108, *111*
  lumbar, osteoporosis and pain in, 104
Spine fusion for tuberculous spondylitis, 48
Splenectomy, Gaucher's disease and, 89
Splenomegaly
  chronic hemolytic anemias and, 119, 120

Splenomegaly—cont'd
  in rickets, 65
  in Still's disease, 204
Spondylitis
  ankylosing, 204
    hereditary ochronosis and, 94, 95-96
    Reiter's syndrome and, 193
  brucellosis and, 43
  "rheumatoid," 204
  rhizomelic, 204
  tuberculous, 48
Spondylolisthesis, 171-172
Spondylolysis, 171
Spondylosis deformans, 197
Sporotrichium, 54
Sporotrichosis, 50, 54
Spotty bones, *28, 29*
Sprue, 65, 69
Staphylococcal infection of joints, 188
Staphylococcus aureus, 38, 188
Stature, loss of, osteoporosis and, 105; *see also*
    Dwarfism
Steatorrhea
  idiopathic, 65
  osteomalacia and, 69
Stenosing tenovaginitis, 159
Steroid therapy, 104, *105*
  bone infarcts and, 165
  histiocytosis X and, 142, 145
Still's disease, 204
Strahlenpilz, 53
Streptococcal infection of joints, 188, *189*
Streptococcal M protein, 205
Streptococcus hemolyticus, 188
Streptomycin, 44, 48
Strontium, bone sarcoma and, 149
Subacute disseminated histiocytosis X, 141-143
Subcutaneous calcification in pseudo-hypoparathy-
    roidism, 84
Subperiosteal hemorrhage, periosteal ossification
    and, 174
Subperiosteal resorption of cortex, hyperparathy-
    roidism and, 81
Subungual exostosis, 175
Sudeck's atrophy, 171
Sulfinpyrazone, 91
Sulfonamides, hypersensitivity reactions to, 206
"Sulfur granules," yellow, in actinomycosis, 53
Suppurative arthritis, 188-189, *189*
Supraspinatous tendon, calcium deposits in, *156,*
    157
Syndromes
  Albright's, 14
  Burnett, 158
  Cushing's, 73, 75, 104
  Debré-de Toni-Fanconi, 66, *66,* 102
  Felty's, 204
  Hurler's, 30-33, *31, 32*
  Lobstein's, 22-24, *25*
  Maffucci's, 19
  milk-alkali, 158
  Milkman's, *68,* 69, *69*
  Reiter's, 193

Syndromes—cont'd
  Turner's osteoporosis and, 104
  van der Hoeve's, 22-24, 25
Synovial chondromatosis, 207-209, *207, 208*
Synovial joints, disorders of, 184-212
  arthritic manifestations of metabolic disorders in, *194, 195,* 196
  chondrocalcinosis in, 207
  chondromatosis of joints in, 207-209, *207, 208*
  chronic hemarthrosis in, 193, 195-196
  chronic villous nonspecific synovitis in, 184-186, *185*
  classification and pathology of nonarticular "rheumatism" in, 206
  hypersensitivity reactions in, 206-207
  infections of joints in, 188-193, *189, 190, 191, 192*
  neurotrophic joint disorders in, 196
  osteoarthritis in, 196-200, *197, 198, 199*
  pigmented villonodular synovitis in, 209-211, *209, 210, 211*
  relapsing polychondritis in, 207
  rheumatoid arthritis in, 200-205, *201, 202, 203*
  systemic connective tissue diseases in, 205-206
  trauma and changes in, 186-188, *186, 187*
Synovitis
  microcrystalline, 91
  pigmented villonodular, 209-211, *209, 210, 211*
    hemarthrosis and, 195
  posttraumatic, differential diagnosis in, 187
  syphilis and, 50
  tuberculous, *191*
  villous
    chronic nonspecific, 184-186, *185*
    rheumatoid arthritis and, *202, 203*
Synovium, joint bodies and, 188
Syphilis
  acquired, 50, *50-51*
  congenital, skeletal hyperostoses and, 49-50, 132
  joint manifestations in, 192-193
  neurotrophic disorders and, 108-109
  skeletal manifestations of, 49-50, *50-51*
Syringomyelia, 108, 113, *113*
Syrinx of spinal cord, neuroarthropathy and, 113
Systematized anomalies of skeletal development; *see* Anomalies of skeletal development, systematized
Systemic connective diseases, joint manifestations in, 205-206
Systemic disorders of mucopolysaccharide metabolism, 97

T

Tabes dorsalis, 108-109
Taboparesis, juvenile, 50
Taenia echinococcus, 54
Teeth
  deformed, syphilis and, 50
  mottling of, fluoride and, 147
Tendon sheaths
  ganglion formation in, 153
  pathologic changes in, 156-159

Tendons
  pathologic changes in, 156-159, *156*
  rupture of, 158-159, *158*
Tenosynovial tuberculosis, 156
Tenosynovitis, pigmented nodular, 157, *210*
Tenovaginitis, stenosing, 159
Teratomas of pineal gland, 77
Tertiary hyperparathyroidism, 102
Tetracycline, 188
Tetracycline derivatives, 44
Thalassemia, 118-119, *120*
Thigh, myositis ossificans and, 173
Thoracic deformity in rickets, 65
Thrombocytopenia, Gaucher's disease and, 87
Thymus, 77
Thyrocalcitonin, 76
Thyroid gland, 76
Thyrotoxicosis, osteoporosis and, 104, 105
Tibia
  congenital pseudoarthrosis of, 163-164, *163*
  Paget's disease and, *127, 128, 129*
Tibial apophysis, Osgood-Schlatter's disease and, 170, *170*
Tibial cortex in congenital pseudoarthrosis, 163
Tibial epiphysis, Blount's disease and, 163
Toe, subungual exostosis and, 175
Tophaceous arthritis, 91
Tophaceous gout, 91-93
Torn menisci, 151, *152,* 196
Torticollis, congenital, 161
Torulosis, 54
Tower skull, spherocytic anemia and, 120
Trabecular architecture, Paget's disease and, 128, *129*
Trace elements, influence of, on skeleton, 97-98
Trauma
  joint changes following, 186-188, *186, 187*
  to knee and lacerated meniscus, 151, *152,* 196
  periosteal ossification and, 174
Traumatic rupture of tendons, 158-159, *158*
Trident hands, 24, *26*
Trigger finger, 159
Tuberculosis
  of joints, 189-190, *190, 191*
  skeletal, *46-47,* 48
  tenosynovial, 156
Tuberculous dactylitis, *46-47,* 48
Tuberculous granulation tissue, 190, *190*
Tuberculous spondylitis, 48
Tuberculous synovitis, *191*
Tubule reabsorption disease, 102
Tumors; *see also* Malignant change
  adrenal cortical, osteoporosis and, 105
  anaplastic, Paget's disease and, 131
  benign giant cell, Paget's disease and, 122
  brown, 79, 81, 82
  as effects of radiation, 149-150
  localized hyperostosis and, 132
  malignant, chronic osteomyelitis and, 44
  of pineal gland, 77
Turmschädel, 120
Turner's syndrome, osteoporosis and, 104

Index

U

Ulceration of gums in vitamin C deficiency, 62
Ulna, monostotic Paget involvement of, *123*
Unicameral bone cyst, 175-180, *176, 177, 178, 179*
Urate deposits in bone in gout, *92, 93*
Urethritis, Reiter's syndrome and, 193
Uric acid levels, serum, in osteogenesis imperfecta, 22
Urinary calcium and phosphorus in hyperthyroidism, 76
Urolithiasis
  Paget's disease and, 125
  primary hyperparathyroidism and, 77

V

Vaccinia, 55
Vaginal epithelium in vitamin A deficiency, 60
van der Hoeve's syndrome, 22-24, *25*
Vanishing bone disease, 171
Vertebra plana, eosinophilic granuloma of bone and, 140-141
Vertebrae; *see also* Spine; Vertebral bodies; Vertebral column
  hereditary ochronosis and, *94, 95*
  slipping, 171
Vertebral bodies; *see also* Vertebrae; Vertebral column
  compression of, osteomalacia and, 69
  flattening or shallowness of, in Morquio's disease, 28
  in osteoporosis, *105*
  Paget's disease and, *126*
  posttraumatic rarefaction of bone and, 171
Vertebral column; *see also* Vertebrae; Vertebral bodies
  aneurysmal bone cyst and, 180, *182*
  displacement of, 171
  eosinophilic granuloma of bone and, *139,* 140-141
  neuroarthropathy and, 108, *111*
  osteoporosis and, 104-105, *106*
Villonodular synovitis, pigmented, 195, 209-211, *209, 210, 211*

Villous synovitis, rheumatoid arthritis and, *202, 203*
Viral infections
  bone changes and, 54-55
  joint manifestations in, 193
Virility, adrenal gland tumors and, 75
Vitamin D in osteoporosis, 105; *see also* Vitamin deficiencies and excesses, skeletal changes in
Vitamin deficiencies and excesses, skeletal changes in, 60-72
  vitamin A
    deficiency in, 60
    excess or poisoning in, 60-61, *61*
  vitamin C deficiency in, 61-64, *62-63*
  vitamin D
    deficiency in, 64-70, *64, 66, 67, 68, 69*
    excess or poisoning in, 70
    infantile vitamin D–deficiency rickets and, 100, *101*
    vitamin D–resistant rickets in, 66, *66*
Volkmann's contracture, 159, *160*
von Bechterew's arthritis, 204
von Recklinghausen's disease, 163
Voorhoeve's disease, 29, *29*

W

Wedge fractures, osteoporosis and, 105
Whipple's disease, osteomalacia and, 69
Wilson's disease, 102
Wryneck, 161

X

Xanthoma tuberosum multiplex, 89-90, *90, 91*
Xerophthalmia, 60

Y

Yaws, 49, *50-51*

Z

Zebra-like effect in osteopetrosis, 21, *22*
Zinc deficiency, 98